100 MARATHONS

100 Marathons
Memories and Lessons from Races Run around the World

Jeffrey Horowitz

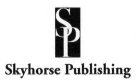

Skyhorse Publishing

Skyhorse Publishing books may be purchased in bulk at special discounts for sales promotion, corporate gifts, fund-raising, or educational purposes. Special editions can also be created to specifications. For details, contact the Special Sales Department, Skyhorse Publishing, 307 West 36th Street, 11th Floor, New York, NY 10018 or info@skyhorsepublishing.com.

Skyhorse® and Skyhorse Publishing® are registered trademarks of Skyhorse Publishing, Inc.®, a Delaware corporation.

Visit our website at www.skyhorsepublishing.com.

10 9 8 7 6 5 4 3 2 1

Paperback ISBN: 978-1-62636-045-7

Library of Congress Cataloging-in-Publication Data
Horowitz, Jeffrey.
My first 100 marathons : 2,620 miles with an obsessive runner / Jeffrey Horowitz. p. cm.
ISBN 978-1-60239-318-9 (hardcover : alk. paper)
1. Marathon running—United States. 2. Marathon running—Training—United States. 3. Long-distance runners—United States—Anecdotes.
4. Horowitz, Jeffrey. I. Title. II. Title: My first hundred marathons.
III. Title: My first one hundred marathons.
GV1065.2.H67 2008
796.42'520973—dc22
2008028945

Printed in the United States of America

To all those who have inspired, challenged, prodded, and pushed me over the years, but most of all to my wonderful wife, Stephanie, for her encouragement and patience, and for bringing Alex Michael into the world.

CONTENTS

Foreword

I sat down to write a book about running, but ended up writing something else.

After running marathons for nearly 20 years, from the Atlantic to the Pacific and across the world from Antarctica to Africa and Asia, there were plenty of good stories to pick from. But as I began to write them down, I discovered that running isn't something that we do; running explains who we are. It shapes the way we view the world and our place in it, and reflects our values, our dreams, and our work ethic.

As the stories unspooled, I found, too, that some of them weren't about running and racing at all, at least not directly. They were about life. There were moments of joy, but also moments of sadness and loss. One reader emailed me saying that the book surprised him because, as he put it, "running books aren't supposed to make you cry." But that's life, isn't it? Running is life is laughter is sorrow is joy is loss. It all becomes one seamless whole.

It would be easy to say that this book is just about my life. That's certainly true, in a way. But I aimed for it to be more than that. It's an invitation. Every runner has a story to tell, and I hoped that my book would resonate with other people, reminding them of their own experiences that were waiting to be shared. I wanted to start a conversation. I wanted people to write me messages saying, "Hey, I loved your book, but let me tell you my story."

I got my wish. I never expected that my book would be popular enough to lead to action figure spin-offs and themed Happy Meals, but I was thrilled to receive a steady stream of emails from people who found my book interesting, entertaining, and thoughtful, and who then had something they wanted to share with me in return. I'm grateful to all of them.

I also found that my editor was right: readers really would be interested in having training and racing advice mixed in along with the stories. Many of the emails I received thanked me for those tips, and asked for follow-up advice. I'm grateful, too, for the chance to help other runners, just as I had been helped so many times with sound advice from my own friends and mentors.

One unexpected question that came from a number of readers, though, was what would I do now that I had reached my goal of running 100 marathons?

I found that perplexing. I would keep running, of course! What else would I do?

Since completing my 100-marathon quest, I've returned to many of my favorite races, but I've also traveled far and wide, running marathons in Florence, Milan, Sydney, and Madrid. I've run a marathon on an indoor 200-meter track in Virginia, and a marathon starting at midnight in the Nevada desert. I've run in a 5-day stage race in the Himalayas in the shadow of Mt. Everest, and in the 3-day TransRockies Run. I also ran in a 100k Ultramarathon in Cairo, Egypt, where I was chased by a pack of wild dogs, had rocks thrown at me by unimpressed teenagers, and was either guarded or threatened by armed villagers, depending on who I asked.

I still seek out these racing adventures, but as my life moved more from Me to We, as my wife and I raise our son, I've slowed down the pace a bit. I still scan the web for interesting new races, and I still haunt those familiar running trails and paths as before, but I find more and more frequently now that I'd rather stay at home with my wife and help our son grow into a young boy than dash off to add another marathon to my list. But still, the marathon continues to have meaning for me. I'm now more than halfway towards my next centennial milestone, and with any luck, I'll be able to continue past that, collecting marathons and adventures for years to come.

More marathons, more stories, more life.

Jeff Horowitz, 2013

Out the Door and Around the Block

There is an old proverb that says a journey of a thousand miles begins with a single step. Sometimes, though, a quick trip to the emergency room begins that way, too.

That was my story. It was 1985. Ronald Reagan was president, New Wave was on the radio, and I had just moved away from home for the first time. I had come down to Washington, D.C., from New York City, for law school. After a rocky start, I found a good roommate, settled in, and acquired a love for my new hometown. I had always been overweight—"husky" was the euphemism the clothing stores seemed to like—but now I had added some new padding around my middle, and I was determined to do something about it. A new body for my new life. Except that as a grad student, I was barely getting by on my meager savings and student loans, living on spaghetti and tuna fish, and using furniture I'd built from of cinder blocks and boards. There wasn't much spare cash for a health club, personal trainer, chef, or a masseuse. But running fit the bill. I already had sneakers and shorts, so all I needed to do was head out the door and begin. Simplicity itself.

I started off with a few slow laps around the block where I lived in Arlington, Virginia. As out of shape as I was, I still immediately recognized how right it felt. I'd played sports as a kid growing up in Queens, New York, but I never excelled; I wasn't what anyone would call a naturally gifted athlete. But I was persistent, which was a trait that cut me out to be a good distance runner. Soon, my runs lengthened into laps around a small park, and then out-and-back runs down the street toward the Potomac River. Reaching my turnaround point, I gazed across the water at the spires of Georgetown University.

In those moments, I was filled with a sense of possibility. Running cleared the day's cobwebs from my mind and focused my thinking, and gave me time and space to sort out anything that was bothering me, or to detach and think of nothing at all. It had also started to reshape my body. Those new extra pounds fell away, taking some of the older, more stubborn fat along with them. Running also made me more aware of my body's needs; I quickly realized that I could only be as good as the fuel I took in, so I started to avoid all of the greasy and sugary foods that had found their way into my diet.

As the months passed, I realized that, little by little, I was actually turning into a real runner. I had never run any races, and I hadn't been on any track teams, but now I felt that I was not just some guy trying to stay in shape. I was an athlete.

If I was going to do this, then, I had to do it right. It was time for me to shelve those ratty old Pro-Keds I'd been running in and upgrade to some real running gear, which is what led me one day to a local sporting-goods store, where I eyed the shoes displayed on the back wall and tried to make sense out of the little information cards that fell out of them. Judging the technology diagrammed on those cards, you would have thought that the shoes had been to the moon and back.

I ended up taking home a pair of gray hi-tech marvels, my first true running shoes. They set me back $69, which seemed wildly extravagant.

As soon as I got home, I laced them up and went out for a run, hoping that I hadn't foolishly wasted my month's eating budget. I didn't expect miracles; all I wanted was that they at least would feel, well, *different.* And they did. Oh, how they did! Suddenly I had spring in my step, and I felt like I could run forever.

Armed with my fancy new shoes, I ran down the street toward the river, but this time I didn't stop. I crossed Key Bridge into D.C., and then followed the river south. I passed the Watergate Hotel and the Kennedy Center for the Performing Arts—a fancy building on the site of an old brewery—and crossed back into Virginia at the next bridge, completing a five-mile loop.

I was hooked. As my runs took me farther, I started wondering what I could do with my newfound love of running. I'd always been the kind of person who hated half steps; once I found a passion for something, I wanted to dive into the deep end of it. It wasn't that I ever needed to prove anything; I just wanted to fully and completely experience whatever it was that intrigued me. And now, that thing was running. I'd have to pursue that passion wherever it led me.

In hindsight, it's also obvious to me now that running provided the perfect counterpoint to sitting at a desk studying law. The mind-numbing tedium of studying left my body aching for some outlet. I didn't understand it at the time, but our bodies need attention and encouragement as much as our minds. They are not meant to be kept quiet, preserved like a specimen in a jar. We are meant to *move.* When we forget that we are not just intellectual, emotional, and spiritual beings, but also animals, we do so at our peril.

As a dedicated runner, then, the obvious next step would be to enter a road race. The idea of having a number pinned to my shirt—a very public declaration that I was a runner, an athlete—was thrilling. But which race? Most new runners start out with a 5K or 10K, but those races were shorter than my training runs. They just couldn't capture my imagination, couldn't give me that intoxicating mix of fear and excitement that I craved. I needed something big.

I knew the answer, of course: the marathon. Growing up, I lived in the shadow of the New York City Marathon. Even though I had never run more than a few miles at a time back then—and even then just barely—I felt that someday I would run that distance. Now, all these years later, the time had come to run a marathon. I would be David, throwing myself against the Goliath of running. If I came out victorious, I would truly understand what it meant to be a runner.

Luckily, one of the best marathons in the country was in my backyard—the Marine Corps Marathon, held the last weekend of every October. It starts at the Iwo Jima Memorial in Arlington, taking runners on a grand tour of D.C. and northern Virginia, circling the Pentagon, the Capitol, the Smithsonian, and the Jefferson and Lincoln Memorials before returning to the Iwo Jima Memorial for the finish. Since its course included some of my new training routes, it was easy for me to imagine running the race. I was nervous, but the more I thought about it, the more reasonable this crazy idea seemed to be.

The mailing of an application is itself a very symbolic and important act. As I wrote the check, sealed the envelope, and dropped it in the mailbox, I felt the solemnity of the moment, and a new seriousness of purpose. *I'm in for it now*, I thought. Even now, decades later, when online registration has mostly replaced the mailing of applications, I pause before clicking the final button that will commit me to a race. *Are you sure you want to do this?* But I knew then—have always known, in those kinds of situations—what I was getting myself into. I wasn't worried about it. It was simply time to get to work.

I began by increasing my weekly mileage, with the goal of building up to a 21-mile run three weeks before the race. In 1986, there wasn't the flood of training advice that runners today have to wade through; there was really very little good information available at all. There was

Jim Fixx's book on running, a few other training books, and a couple of running magazines. I read as much as I could, and more or less sorted my way through it by trial and error.

Sometimes this involved more error than I liked to admit. Once, after a good 15-mile run, I decided to run 15 miles every day, on the reasonable—though entirely wrong—assumption that if a little is good, more must be better. After a week of this, my muscles ached and I was tired to the bone. Obviously, my 15-mile-a-day plan wasn't a good idea.

Despite my blunders and setbacks, my training advanced, and finally I completed my last long run. I had met my training goal. I was ready for the marathon! Elated, I went on a short celebration run the next day with my roommate. We followed a horse trail into the woods—not my usual route—and early into the run I rolled my foot on a rock. I felt a sharp pain in my ankle, and I knew instantly that I had sprained it badly. I considered stopping, but I thought that managing pain was part of being a marathoner, so I decided to keep running.

Bad idea. There's often a very fine line between bravery and stupidity and on that Sunday morning in October 1986, I crossed it. After running 6 more miles, I made it back to my room, slumped in an easy chair, gently removed my running shoes, and inspected the damage. My ankle had turned as dark as thunderclouds, and was quickly swelling up to double its normal size. I phoned my girlfriend Kathleen and quietly, humbly, asked if she could drive me to the emergency room. Kathleen had no love of running, but she knew from the sound of my voice that this was serious. She came right over.

My short little celebration run had landed me on crutches. I was out of the marathon. I had thrown all my hard work out the window. I had blown my once-in-a-lifetime opportunity. I was devastated.

The death of a dream is a sad and painful thing. Eventually, I reconciled myself to my loss, and focused on just returning to a regular running routine. Once again, though, I demonstrated my capacity for stupidity by rushing my recovery and reinjuring my ankle. Once. Twice. Three times. Little by little, I managed to parlay a simple sprain into a six-month layoff.

Finally, showing a glimmer of wisdom, I left my ankle alone until it felt completely healed, and then left it alone some more. Eventually, I was able to return to a regular, pain-free, modest running routine.

As the weeks went by, though, I found myself thinking again about the marathon. It was like an old lover you swore you'd never call again, but whose number you kept. I began increasing my weekly mileage, waiting for the pain to come, but it never did. Finally, one day I wrote another check and sealed another envelope. I was going back to the Marine Corps Marathon.

In the final weeks before the race I was cautious to a fault, refusing to run off-road, step on cracks, or walk under ladders. I was rewarded by making it to the race day healthy and whole. Before the race even started, I had already accomplished my goal.

There were things that I still had left to learn, however. As I walked to the starting line near the Iwo Jima Memorial, I saw a woman standing just a few feet from the roadway, near a tree. She was carefully holding back her shorts to one side as she crouched slightly in the direction of the tree. It took me a moment to realize what she was doing. She was peeing. Right there, in front of 13,000 runners and their families and friends. Even more startling, though, was the fact that no one around her seemed the least bit surprised. She could have been blowing her nose for all they cared.

It was a revelation. I wasn't yet familiar with running culture, with the fact that runners are endlessly fascinated with their bodies—how they work, how they look, what goes into them, and most importantly, what comes out and when. And they were not the least bit shy about discussing all these issues with anyone at any time. Remember: I had done most of my training alone at that point, so I was like a feral child, a Tarzan among socialized runners.

Then the starting cannon roared—a Marine Corp Marathon tradition—and I had no more time to think about such things. The crowd surged forward. We began to run, and then suddenly, inexplicably, came to a full stop. Bodies crashed into one another. After a few moments of awkward shuffling, the crowd moved forward again, and we were able to settle into a regular running pace.

I was confused. What had just happened? There was open road in front of us. Why the sudden traffic jam? I didn't know it at the time, but that stop-and-go phenomenon happens in almost every big race. And I still don't know why. But I've learned not to let it bother me.

I ran cautiously, hoping to save enough energy to get me through the final few miles. We ran south to the Pentagon before returning north and crossing Key Bridge into D.C. We ran past the historic row houses and shops of Georgetown, and along the riverfront to the Lincoln Memorial, where we turned eastward toward the Smithsonian museums and the Capitol. I thought about how this route must seem for the out-of-town runners; even as a resident, I often have moments—as I did during the race—where I'm startled by how beautiful D.C. is.

I passed the halfway point at the U.S. Capitol feeling surprisingly strong. With 13 miles behind me, I decided to take a calculated risk—I picked up the pace. Streaking downhill past the Smithsonian museums, I passed the Jefferson Memorial and turned south toward lonely Hains Point, a pointy spit of land—landfill, actually—that juts out into the Potomac River.

This would be the make-or-break point for many runners. Hains Point brought with it miles 19 and 20 of the race, where the dreaded Wall lurked. If a runner had not properly prepared his or her body during training to burn fat, then it would be somewhere around this point where the supplies of blood sugar in the body—glycogen—would be used up. When that happens, a runner feels like someone just cut his or her power cord. Even well-trained runners who don't face this problem still find this stretch of road difficult because so many miles have been conquered, but there are still so many miles yet to come. This is the point where mental toughness weighs in. It's no wonder that veteran runners say the marathon is really two races: the first 20 miles, and the last 6.2.

I didn't know all of this at the time, which was probably a good thing, since I couldn't worry about something I wasn't expecting. But as I approached the turnaround at the tip of Hains Point, I felt my energy wane and my willpower slip. I was suddenly so tired of running.

Then I saw him. Or rather, heard him. A lone fan, standing beside his open car trunk at the tip of Hains Point, was blasting the theme from *Rocky* on his car stereo. Suddenly, adrenaline surged through my veins, and I felt new life in my tired legs as I followed the course back north for the final few miles to the finish line.

Before I could claim my finisher's medal, however, there was the 14th Street Bridge, a long, wide, rolling overpass that would take us from D.C. to Virginia. I later learned to call this stretch the Anvil of God, since, on a warm day, the sun can pour heat down on a runner along this stretch with unrivaled cruelty.

On this day, though, I had come too far to be denied, and I conquered that last obstacle and then raced the final few miles toward the finish line at the Iwo Jima Memorial. I passed the final mile marker— Mile 26!—and followed the course up a short, steep incline toward the memorial. Spectators massed along the retaining fence cheered as I followed the course as it circled the memorial, eager for a glimpse of that glorious finish line.

But where was it? Those final two-tenths of a mile seemed to stretch on forever. But finally, there it was: the finish line. I crossed it, and turned toward one of the marines to accept my finisher's medal. "Outstanding," he said. And I had to admit, it was.

I had run the second half 15 minutes faster than the first half, an impressive negative split, as I later learned to call it. I felt both brilliantly alive and bone tired, something I'd never before experienced, but that I completely enjoyed. I even liked the soreness that overtook my legs over the next few days. My friends were horrified watching me hobble downstairs backward, but I knew that every ache meant that I had faced my fear and doubt and won. I had run a marathon.

Having reached that milestone, I turned toward a few others that were on my calendar. In 1988, I graduated from law school, passed the bar exam, and began working as an attorney with the federal government. Instead of making D.C. a quick stopover, I was settling down as a permanent resident. And instead of being a distraction from my studies, running became my lifestyle. Perhaps if I spent less time in front of a computer, I wouldn't have become so devoted to it. Or maybe I was genetically predisposed to run. Either way, I found myself figuring out how to fit my running into my new work schedule. I woke up before dawn to run, brought my gear to the office for a quick lunchtime workout, and ran on weekends. Whatever it took, I made it work.

Three years later, I ran the Marine Corps Marathon again, no longer burdened with a fear of the unknown, but instead looking for another hit of that exhilarated/exhausted feeling. After another successful run, I turned homeward, toward New York City. I was finally ready to check off that boyhood goal.

On race morning, I stood shoulder to shoulder with 20,000 other runners in Staten Island, at the foot of the Verrazano Bridge. The gun went off, and we all surged up the mile-long climb to the apex of the bridge, jostling for a little elbow room along the way. After cresting, I found myself warmed up and energized for the mile-long descent. It was the fastest mile I'd ever run. And I still had 24 more miles to go. I quickly realized how monumentally stupid I'd just been, and how I'd pay dearly for it later in the race.

I settled down into a slower pace and made my way through Brooklyn and Queens, and then climbed the Queensboro Bridge to Manhattan. As I descended on the far side—at a comfortable pace, this time!—I began to hear a mysterious low roar. I was almost on the Manhattan side, but I still couldn't see where the noise was coming from. Then I saw it: a solid mass of people, five or six deep, straining the barricades, screaming like they had lost their minds. I was dumbstruck.

The party continued up First Avenue, as people lined the streets, hung out windows, crowded onto balconies, and stood on rooftops, all cheering like mad. I felt like an astronaut in a parade. It shot a bolt of lightning into me. I ran effortlessly up toward Harlem.

That's where my earlier foolishness hit me. This time I was the one who felt as though someone had cut my power cord. I was reduced to walking. Suddenly, a huge man jumped out of the crowd and rushed toward me. I braced myself, but he just yelled, "I didn't come out here to see you walk!" Believe me, I was back to running in no time flat!

From there, it was on to the Bronx, into neighborhoods that I had never seen in all my years living in New York. Then it was time for the homestretch down Fifth Avenue and into Central Park. My mother and younger sister were waiting for me near the finish line, and had talked other bystanders into cheering for me as I came into view, but I was so focused on the finish line that I never heard a thing. No matter. Just knowing they were there, watching for me and cheering me onward, gave me the extra strength I needed.

Finishing that race meant a lot to me. It taught me that I could overcome adversity during a race, and also that I had a lot yet to learn about running this thing.

In March of 1993, I ran my fourth marathon, in Virginia Beach. After the race, in the hotel corridor, I met an older runner who told me that he had just run his thirty-fifth marathon. I was astonished.

The number seemed impossible, like Joe DiMaggio's consecutive-game hitting streak. I was sure that this guy was a different breed of runner.

I expected to feel tired after the Virginia Beach marathon, but instead, I craved more. There was something about the marathon that called to me, that captured my imagination, that left me feeling a sense of accomplishment like I'd experienced nowhere else. I wasn't sure if it was a good idea to run another marathon so soon—I hadn't heard of anyone else doing something like that—but I felt fresh and strong, and was certainly motivated, so I ran the Pittsburgh Marathon two months later, where the scorching heat reduced me to walking most of the last few miles. My suffering there was alleviated by the sight of one late-night reveler in leather pants and boots, who, after stumbling out his door and squinting at the bright daylight, looked at all the runners streaming past and asked someone, "Where are they all going?"

I ran two more marathons that same year, still electrified by the experience. Like a child who's discovered how to walk, I was amazed at what my body could now do. It was as if I'd walked through a doorway into a brand-new, beautiful room that I hadn't known was there. I even began to earn a reputation at work as being an avid marathoner; I became known as *that running guy*.

The marathons then came in bunches, like a blizzard following a few errant snowflakes. I ran six in 1994, including one in Philadelphia, where I found myself desperate at one point to relieve myself, but without a Porta-Jon or bush in sight. Spectators lined the streets, but I had little choice but to use a light post as my bathroom stall. Looking over to my left, I saw a policeman. He just looked the other way. This road racing was a funny business.

By 1995 people had begun calling me "obsessed," but I thought of myself as just being enthusiastic, and I continued running and racing. I traveled back and forth across the continent, and overseas as well. In 1998, in Madison, Wisconsin, I reached marathon number 35, and I realized that I was now like the older runner I had met a few years earlier in Virginia Beach. Like him, I was now a different breed of runner.

But what kind of runner was I now? I had proven beyond any doubt that I could run a marathon, and yet the marathon distance still intrigued me. Rather than slaking my thirst for racing, each marathon left me wanting more. I knew that I could simply keep running and racing, but that alone wouldn't be enough. I had entered my first marathon because I needed a goal to focus my training. Now I needed a similar goal to focus my racing. I had proven to myself that although I might not be the fastest runner in the field, I was one of the most durable. So my challenge would be to find out exactly how durable I was. If thirty-five marathons once amazed me, what would be a suitable goal now?

100 marathons. As soon as I thought of it, I knew that I had the right answer. Even if it was an arbitrary number, it was beautiful. It seemed complete. Ninety-nine marathons cried out for one more; 101 marathons seemed a stop on the way toward another goal. But 100 was perfect. It was also a number that would, in its audacity, seem insane even to other athletes. Totaled up in miles, it described a course heading west from my home in Washington, D.C., all the way to Carson City, Nevada. It was a feat of running that most people couldn't imagine, but it was something that I really felt that I could do. The thought of it also scared and exhilarated me, which meant, of course, that it was just the kind of challenge I was looking for.

In fact, as I discovered, I wasn't the first person to take on and beat such a challenge. Still, the club of people who have run 100 marathons is a pretty select one, and even if that weren't true—even if hundreds of thousands of other runners across the globe had done it—it was not something *I* had done. And that was the point. Ultimately, it was going to be a challenge not of the human spirit and body, but of *my* spirit and body. And so I committed myself to it.

Then, seemingly way too soon, it happened. It actually took eighteen years, but it happened. One hundred marathons. 2,620 miles of racing. Finished.

Here are the memories and lessons of those eighteen years of marathon racing. My first 100 marathons. Compressed within these pages are the joys and agonies of all those long miles, and, I hope, some of the knowledge that came from making a habit of pushing myself beyond pain and fear and doubt.

When I talk about my marathons, I feel like a child who can't wait to show his birthday gift to his friends. "See this? Isn't it the coolest thing you've ever seen?" After almost two decades, I think it still is, and by the time you've reached the end of this journey, I hope you'll see why.

Running Tip #1

Getting Started

- *Get proper gear.* Buy shoes in a proper running store, where they can identify your particular needs. And avoid cotton clothing; cotton stays wet and makes you colder if you're cold and hotter if you're hot.
- *Warm up.* Start each run with a 5-minute walk or slow jog. Running too hard too soon will only make for a miserable run.
- *Breathe smoothly.* Find a pace that allows you to talk while running. Runners who run out of breath don't run very long.
- *Stay relaxed.* Keep your shoulders low, and swing your arms smoothly, with your hands near your upper hip.
- *Don't overstride.* Your foot should land directly under your body.
- *Don't be too ambitious!* Keep your mileage increases to no more than 10 percent from week to week.

Why Run the Marathon? First Lap

Looking back, I could see that once I put on my first pair of running shoes and set out down the street, it was probably inevitable that I would want to run a marathon. Like a Little League baseball player dreaming of the major leagues, distance runners dream of the marathon.

It didn't necessarily have to be that way—I'm told that there are runners out there who are content to do their training and never pin on a race number. Regular training, as opposed to racing, brings all the proven benefits of weight control, cardiovascular health, and improved emotional outlook, and all with as little work as three sessions of 20–30 minutes a week. And many runners who choose to race are often content to just run 5Ks and 10Ks. But that wasn't good enough for me, or for almost a half-million other people in the United States every year who are drawn to the marathon. Why? At some level, it isn't good enough to just say that it seemed like a good challenge, that it felt right, that it was hard but fun.

It's a simple question, really, so there should be a simple answer: Why run the marathon?

Perhaps the answer is in our desire to be part of something bigger than ourselves, to connect with history and become a part of it. The marathon, after all, is the most famous and storied of all footraces. Here's the original story, in a thumbnail sketch, taken straight from Herodotus (more or less): Sometime around 490 BC, Darius the Great of Persia amassed a huge army and moved to conquer each of the Greek city-states, which had not yet united into a single power. The cities fell one by one, and soon only Athens and Sparta remained independent.

Darius landed some 30,000 soldiers at the plains of Marathon and prepared to attack Athens. Athens gathered a force of 10,000 soldiers to meet them under the leadership of Athenian general Miltiades, who immediately sent a runner named Phidippides to Sparta, some 150 miles distant, to ask for help. The Spartans were celebrating a religious holiday, and would only send warriors once the festival ended five days later. Phidippides raced back and relayed the news to Miltiades, who decided to strike alone before the Persians became fully prepared. The Athenians flanked the Persians and then encircled them, hacking their way through toward the Persian center. Once the carnage had ended, Darius's army had suffered some 6,400 casualties, while Miltiades had lost a scant 192 men. More or less.

News of the victory was delivered by a *hemerodromoi*—an "all-day runner." And that was the end of that. Except that centuries later, in the retelling, it was Phidippides who raced the 25 miles from the battlefield to Athens, shouted *"Nenikékamen!"*—we are victorious!"—and then dropped dead.

More or less.

Well, the battle certainly happened, as a large burial mound on the modern plains of Marathon silently confirms. And runners were certainly used as messengers. As for the rest, well, we'll never know for sure.

Now flash forward: the modern Olympic Games were being held in 1896 in Athens, and among the events planned was a 25-mile footrace called a marathon, held in commemoration of Phidippides's legendary run. The race ended with a dramatic and rousing victory for the Greek runner Spiridon Louis. Witnessing the first Olympic Games was a young Bostonian who was so enamored of the marathon that upon returning home, he convinced his athletic club to host a similar marathon race. Thus was born the Boston Marathon, the oldest annually held marathon in the world. But the marathon race wasn't yet a set distance; it wasn't yet the race we know today.

By 1908, the Olympic movement was firmly established, and the Games were being held in London. The royal family, apparently impressed by the fortitude of the distance runners, wanted to witness the race finish from the royal box. Accommodating their wishes added another mile and 385 yards to the 25-mile race distance. And that's how we ended up with the strange total of 26.2 miles for the marathon race.

The marathon, as an established race, is now over a century old. We have seen barefoot champions and computer chips in racers' shoes, and the erosion of racial and gender biases. We have also seen record times drop to seemingly inhuman levels, with the current world's best mark at 2 hours, 4 minutes, 26 seconds for men and 2 hours, 15 minutes, 25 seconds for women.[1]

---

1 These records were set by Haile Gebrsellasie of Ethiopia in the 2007 Berlin Marathon and Paula Radcliffe of Great Britain in the 2003 London Marathon.

Amazing stories. Captivating figures. Triumph, elation, tears, and disappointment. It's all there. Perhaps, then, we marathoners race to become part of this great tradition, to become part of an unbroken line of history stretching back to those brave Athenians, to share in the glory.

Perhaps, except that most modern marathoners probably don't know all of this history when they toe the line on race day, and in truth, it would have little impact on their choice to race a marathon even if they did. And glory? No. Except for the lucky few elite runners, modern marathoners do not race for fame or fortune. We toil in obscurity, part of the mass of bobbing heads that fill a city's streets on a Sunday morning once a year. Our friends and family will tire of congratulating us after several days have gone, and our names and finishing times will eventually be lost to history.

So, again, why run the marathon?

Maybe the answer is not in the history of the race, but in the moment, in the here and now of conquering the racecourse. Few of us ever find ourselves enjoying the adulation of the crowds, and having thousands of people screaming encouragement and calling your name is an adrenaline rush of the first magnitude. That would certainly get most people out of bed in the morning.

Some people misunderstand the attraction of cheering, though. An administrative assistant in my office once decided to write a short piece about my running for our newsletter. I started by explaining to him the thrill of Boston and New York. During everyday life, I told him, you rarely know exactly where you stand. You might be doing great at work and in your relationship, or you might be doing badly, but most often it's hard to tell. Life is filled with mixed signals, and anything can change in a second, often with little explanation, and no one cheers you on if you do the right thing. But when you run a marathon, life is wonderfully and beautifully simple. You run 26.2 miles as fast as you can, and you get a medal if you finish. Along the way you have hundreds or thousands of people telling you what a great job you're doing and how great you look. What's not to love about that?

My interviewer nodded appreciatively and diligently took notes. When he left my office, I felt like an evangelist who had just brought someone new into the flock. *He gets it,* I thought.

Then the newsletter came out, and I quickly turned to his article. "Jeff is going to run the Boston Marathon this month," it began. "He said he does it for the attention." Ugh.

But while the cheers of the crowd are a good motivation for a great many people, a few hours of cheering hardly seems a good return on the months of sacrifice and effort that preceded it. Cheers also cannot fully explain my own marathon odyssey, because few of my marathons attract runners by the tens of thousands. Some of them cannot attract even 100 racers. Instead of being cheered by hundreds of thousands of spectators and fans at these races, I'm often only quietly observed only by a few hardy volunteers shivering by their refreshment tables. On those days, far from the boisterous crowds, the question remains: Why the marathon?

The failure to be able to explain my running passion became a problem for me. The more I was asked the question, the more I realized that I needed an answer, if only for my own peace of mind. I came to fear that perhaps I wasn't running *toward* something, so much as I was running *away* from something. One day I watched a report on television about a man who overcame his addiction to drugs and alcohol by running a marathon every weekend. The interviewer marveled at the amazing transformation, but I wasn't so impressed. It sounded to me only that the man had traded one set of addictions for another. I had seen people like that, and the results were never good. Eventually, the wheels would come off, and some debilitating injury would end their marathon streak. Usually the person would then lurch off in another direction, and become addicted to something else. I felt that my own enthusiasm was much different, but how could I be sure?

What I needed were some tests, some indicators that I had not wandered off onto dangerous ground. I found one while racing in St. Louis in 1997. During the course of 26.2 miles, you tend to notice the other runners around you. It's not uncommon for strangers to congratulate one another at the finish line, or to strike up a conversation and offer encouragement during the race to pass the time. In St. Louis, I realized that the man next to me had matched me stride for stride over several miles.

"Nice pace," I told him. "You're looking strong."

"Thanks," he replied. "I need to be fast. I told my wife that I wouldn't do this anymore. She thinks I'm out getting the newspaper."

I'm no marriage counselor, but even I could see trouble there.

From that exchange, I spotted a potential test: I would simply ask whether I had ever tried to hide my running. Although the answer wouldn't say much about why I was running, it would, hopefully, prove that whatever the reason was, it wasn't a bad one.

I probed my memory, and found my answer: I hadn't lied about my racing.

I then asked myself a second question: had I ever forced myself to run? Sure, there were some days where it was a bit tough getting out the door, but I generally looked forward to my runs, and enjoyed them. There was a moment in just about every run where I felt strong and eternal; not exactly the mythical "runner's high," but a comforting sense of well-being that made all the difficult parts of the run worthwhile. Skeptics say it's simply the result of an endorphin and adrenaline cocktail that my body concocts for me, but that seemed such a spiteful way of describing it, like describing love as a product of certain glandular secretions. When I feel it, it feels great, and that's good enough for me. Of all of life's great pleasures—sex, a great meal, a glorious sunset— a good run has to be near the top.

Such pleasure hardly ever comes without a price, however. If the pleasure of running is truly chemical, it's possible to become addicted to those chemicals. Evidence of such addiction isn't hard to find; many runners insist on hitting the roads despite aching joints and strained muscles. It seems like they had somehow lost sight of the fact that running is supposed to make them feel better, not worse. It's important to be dedicated enough to train hard. However, as I learned—the hard way—it's even more important to be dedicated enough to know when to stop.

I discovered the next test in my third attempt at the Marine Corps Marathon. After finding success in 1987, I decided to try again the following year. I had a difficult training cycle, though, and had dramatically cut back on my running in order to relieve an ache in my knees. My injury disappeared, but as I stood at the starting line before the race, I was nervous that my sacrifice left me unprepared for the race.

I flew through the early miles in the race, and I began to think that I had worried needlessly. But the first lesson of the marathon is not to put too much stock in how you feel at any one moment, since there is plenty of time for things to change. Sure enough, an hour later I was struggling badly. Like a car that has run out of gas, but is still rolling, I shuffled onward toward the finish. Doubt crept into my thinking for the first time, and I began to realize that I would soon have to make a tough decision.

At mile 17 I looked down at my feet, and saw that they were hardly moving, with 9 miles still left to go. I was exhausted, and I suddenly knew that the time had come. I dropped out of the race. I stepped over to the curb and just stopped. It was an odd sensation. Just stepping off the course is a temptation that nips at the heels of every runner who finds himself or herself in distress, but the desire to stay on the course is so great that most of us would rather risk a complete breakdown and injury than take those few steps to the side. But when I did it, it felt as though I no longer even had a choice. I was through, and I knew it. To confirm that point, my muscles stiffened and cramped as soon as I hit the grass.

I should have been upset about my failure, but I wasn't. I knew I had fought as valiantly as I could, but that it was simply not my day. Elite runners drop out of races all the time to save their bodies from unnecessary punishment. But even as I was heading home, I began to analyze why it had happened. Being at peace with my decision to drop out didn't mean that I ever wanted to repeat that experience.

In the years since that day, I have looked back on that DNF (Did Not Finish) as a benchmark of sorts. It was proof that I knew when it was time to quit. Since then, every time I pass mile 17 in a race, I think of that failure, and remind myself that I would always struggle to run the best race that I could, but that in the end, I would not push myself into the danger zone out of sheer stubbornness. I knew that as much as I wanted to finish every race that I entered, I would never be unmindful of the cost. After overcoming injuries and setbacks, I would not sell my running future for a fleeting moment of personal glory on race day. I would not force myself to run.

Still, simply refraining from lying about my racing and avoiding injuries hardly sounds like a ringing endorsement for a lifestyle choice. I was hoping for something that would be a little more useful, that would get to the heart of my running. Ultimately, I found it, and it was a simple thing.

Crossing the finish line, as I had explained to countless people, was a wonderful, life-changing experience, and its glory is never diminished by the number of times I've done it. If anything, my earlier DNF only made each marathon finish that much more precious to me, since I had been forced to realize how much could go wrong in preparing for and racing a marathon. I came to realize that if ever I should cross a finish line and feel disappointed over my time and my performance, the marathon would no longer be a transcendent event for me. It would have lost its meaning, and devolved into drudgery and work. When that happened, I knew that it would be time for me to quit.

So far, though, that day had not yet come, and each marathon finish was a life-affirming event for me, whether I ran my best times or my worst, because in each marathon I did my best, and that was cause enough for celebration.

With those thoughts in mind, I gave myself a clean bill of mental health, reassured that I was not running for the wrong reasons. But still, I had not really answered the question why. But why does anyone do anything? Why do painters paint and singers sing? I realized that I would not be able to answer this question all at once, so I put it away to ponder another time, and went out for a run.

A New Quest

By the end of 1995, I had run eighteen marathons, but my life had changed quite a bit. As an attorney with the National Labor Relations Board, I protected employees' rights to act together to improve their working conditions. It was an interesting job, exposing me to stories from a great number of people from all walks of life, and giving me an opportunity to help people who had been treated unfairly. But as much satisfaction as I got from that job, I was still enthralled by my running. At work, it was frustrating to see how many people I couldn't help—or couldn't help enough—and there were days when I wondered how much I had really accomplished.

With running, however, my achievements were clear, and the joy I took in my running wasn't tempered by any misgivings or compromises. Little by little, running spilled over into all the corners of my life; even the drawers in my office were filled with energy bars and running clothes.

And I had still not yet become bored of the marathon. I had braved an arctic cold front in Delaware that brought windchill temperatures below zero and froze sweat into icicles hanging from runners' headbands and caps. I had completed marathons in eleven different states, from Virginia to Nevada, plus D.C. It occurred to me that with a little organization, I could run a marathon in every state. The thought quickly settled comfortably in my mind. It was an elegantly simple and daunting challenge. Fifty states, fifty marathons. An added bonus to my goal of running 100 marathons, there for the taking.

As it turned out, just as with my 100-marathon goal, I hadn't been the first person to imagine this quest, either. There was actually an informal club of runners who had set this goal for themselves, and some of them were even working on their second tally. Rather than feeling diminished by this fact, however, I felt comforted. Nothing confirms our sanity more than finding out that there are people out there crazier than ourselves. Membership in the club was open to runners who had completed marathons in ten different states. I was eligible, so I joined the club. I was now an official marathon lunatic.

During the six years that I'd been racing, I also had seen my best time, my Personal Record time, drop from 3 hours, 45 minutes in my first marathon, to 3 hours, 35 minutes. Ten minutes may not sound like much, but it felt like a monumental achievement to me.

My dream for the marathon, my fantasy goal, was to qualify for the Holy Grail of road racing, the Boston Marathon. Boston was special to me not only for its storied history, but also for its elitism; it was the only marathon in the country for which you had to prequalify. There are no slow, novice racers in Boston, at least not officially, because having a race number itself means that you have already finished a marathon in qualifying time. The required times vary according to age and gender, as explained on the race Web site. I was in the most challenging group: men under 35 years of age. To toe the line in Boston, I would have to run a marathon in 3 hours 10 minutes or less. That was 25 minutes faster than I had run a marathon in six years of racing. Impossible. Or so I thought.

Qualifying is not actually the only way to the start line for the Boston Marathon. The Boston Athletic Association donates a certain number of race numbers to designated charities, which give them to runners who have met a designated fundraising goal. I was so sure that I would never qualify for the race that I managed to get a number this way. So I ran Boston, but I did not have the "Boston Marathon experience." I hadn't qualified, and I didn't have the kind of speed or toughness to run Boston the way it deserved to be run. Rather than a race, my marathon there felt more like a long training run. It just didn't feel right. I swore to myself that if I ever lined up at the start of another Boston Marathon, it would be because I had earned it, and deserved to be there. Until that happened, in my mind, I had never really run the race.

I kept running, and my times did improve. I posted 3:21:28 in Chicago in October 1995, and then 3:19:41 in the Mayor's Midnight Marathon in Anchorage Alaska in June 1996. That race wasn't held at midnight, as its name promised, but it might as well have been. There really isn't any darkness in Alaska in June. There is daylight, twilight, then daylight again. It was a confusing place for someone from "the Lower 48." There were none of the telltale signs of gathering evening. At one point I realized that it was late evening only because all of the stores had closed. Apart from that, it looked like high noon.

I couldn't help having a bit of fun with this; I called my mother and told her that I was calling from a pay phone in a park in the dead of night. Being a native New Yorker, Mom feared the worst. "Get out of there!" she told me, her voice rising. "Don't worry, Mom. I'm just watching a softball game right now, under clear blue skies."

I returned from Alaska still nine minutes from qualifying for Boston. It might as well have been nine hours for all it mattered. I was sure that I had pushed my body to its limit; it had gone about as fast as it would ever go.

Then I discovered track workouts. I had always trained alone, but I knew that running didn't have to be that way. I found out about a running club in D.C. that held track workouts every Wednesday at Georgetown University, and one day after work I showed up at the track, curious and eager. By the time it was over, I felt like I had stepped from the black-and-white world of Kansas into the splendor of Oz. I had discovered speed work.

Speed work, also called interval training, conditions the body to run faster by alternating hard repeats of shorter distances with slower recovery laps. Done correctly, it avoids the injuries that come with added stress from hard running, while making the most of the beneficial adaptations caused by hard running. It was as different from running long miles as riding a supercharged motorcycle is from taking a leisurely drive in the country.

I loved it. On the first day I showed up for training, I was near the back of the pack during the workout, but in the following weeks I slowly moved up toward the front. We ran different workouts every week—quarter-mile intervals, half miles, miles. Each one was an adventure. Ironically, the trick was not running too hard, since sprinting improves short distance speed, but doesn't prepare the body to run faster for longer distances. It took wisdom and experience to know how fast to run, and little by little, I learned.

The coach who called out our weekly workouts assured us that speed work would not only improve our race times but also familiarize us with pacing, as we learned to associate given effort levels with particular clock times. If I had any doubts about this claim, they were dispelled when I ran with a woman who told me her exact goal for each repeat, and then proceeded to run each interval within a second or two of her goal, without ever looking at her watch. She did it by feel alone.

I was impressed. That was the kind of runner I wanted to be.

I met other runners as well at the track: men and women, old and young, fast and, well, less fast. I joined them for food and beer after the workouts, and met them for long Sunday morning runs. There was Camilla, Yvonne, Stewart, Darryl, and two Beths, both of whom were fast runners. I was discovering that running didn't have to be a solitary sport; there was a running *community*.

One day on the track, I tried to block out the discomfort of hard running by thinking about West Virginia. A marathon was being held there that coming Sunday, and I was debating whether I wanted to drive out there to run it. In addition to adding to my overall marathon total, racing in West Virginia would also add to my total of states, since I hadn't entered a marathon there yet. That was the positive side. I would have to drive out there alone to do it, though. That was the negative.

By the time the workout was over, I still hadn't decided what to do. As I stretched and gathered up my gear, another runner told me in passing that he was debating running a marathon that weekend himself. It was June, when few marathons are held because of the heat. Could he be thinking about West Virginia? He was. Would he be interested in going out there together and splitting the driving? He was. That's how I met Dave Harrell.

Dave was more than twenty years older than me. He had come to marathoning later in life, but like me, had taken to it with a passion. He had run a dozen or so marathons, all over the mid-Atlantic and Northeast. He ran with an easy, gliding style, an economy of effort that enabled him to win or place in his age group in many of the races in which he competed.

Dave, however, differed from me in one important respect: his racing strategy. Not one for subtlety, Dave started each race with the intent to run as fast as he could for as long as he could. While most runners start off conservatively and then try to maintain or even increase their speed over the miles, Dave liked to jump out in front early, which he usually paid for with great suffering in the final few miles. It was an unorthodox style, strange to see and difficult to match, uncommon in a runner with Dave's experience. But that was how Dave liked to run, and he wasn't going to change.

The race in West Virginia was called the Ridge Runner, and true to its name, it started with two daunting climbs in the first mile up a ridge, with another long ascent late in the race, and a fast, painful descent at the end. At the crack of the starter's gun, I was surprised to see Dave take off like a bat out of hell. I had thought we might run together, at least for a while, but upon seeing the road rise up in front of me, I decided to let him go, and concentrated on hauling myself up to the top of the ridge. As the race wore on, I found myself feeling stronger, as I usually did at some point midway through my races, and I picked up my pace. It was a beautiful course, and I enjoyed the views all the way through to the end. I flew down the final descent and crossed the finish line, and finally found Dave, who had already crossed the line before me. As I soon learned, he had only crossed it some 41 seconds before I did.

Dave and I didn't know each other well at this point, but that didn't stop us from talking trash. I thought it was obvious that if I had known that he was less than a minute in front of me, I would have sped up and caught him. Unbelievably, Dave insisted that if he knew I was right behind him, he would have sped up and left me in the dust. By the time we made it back to our hotel, we had decided that there was only one way to resolve our dispute: a 40-yard dash. Never mind that we just ran a difficult marathon. Our competitive fires were lit, and there was no other way to douse them.

So, still wearing our race clothing, now whitened with a salt residue from our sweat, we marked out the course in front of the hotel: from here to that second streetlight. *Go!* I ran as fast as I could, but I was horrified to see Dave pull a step in front of me. Laughing and yelling, I lunged forward and grabbed at his singlet, but he evaded me and made it to the finish first. Again. Grrrrr! No hard feelings, though; it had all been in fun, and we went into our hotel to clean up and check out.

On the ride home, and later at the track, Dave and I talked about our race goals. I suggested to Dave that given his past marathoning experience, and his ambitious plans for the future, all it would take for him to also complete the fifty states would be a bit of organization and planning. With his volume of racing, if we timed it right, Dave and I might also reach 100 marathons together. Dave rolled it around in his mind for a moment, then grinned. I had found a racing partner.

I don't know what drove Dave to run with such dedication. It wasn't something we ever spoke about. Sometimes those kinds of questions are the hardest to answer; I still wasn't even exactly sure why I took to long-distance running like I had. At the least, it was a good balance to the hours I spent at a desk. I've heard it said that running is like meditation, since the rhythm of the legs and the breathing can lull one into a quiet, thought-free state. I've experienced that, but I've also experienced moments of deep, focused thought, where I worked through problems and issues that have arisen in my life. Perhaps my love of running came from one of these things, or perhaps it came from them all. Or, perhaps, it came from something else entirely. I couldn't exactly say.

I don't know if Dave wondered about these things. If he did, he never told me. We did most of our communication with our legs, over hundreds and hundreds of miles. We both knew, without ever saying it aloud, that each of us had recognized that there was something perfect about the marathon, something that made it one of the most important things in our lives. We understood this about each other. There was nothing more that needed to be said. Any other questions that I had, I would have to answer on my own.

Running Tip #2

Ten-Week Speed Program

It's been said that there are as many running programs as there are coaches. Here's mine. Give it a chance, and remember to do a 1-mile warm-up and cooldown.

- Week 1—4 X 880m (half-mile) @ 10K race pace/moderately hard (15–20 seconds faster than marathon race pace), with a 440m slow recovery between each repeat
- Week 2—6 X 880m @ 10K race pace/moderately hard, with a 440m recovery
- Week 3—440m (quarter mile), 880m, 1320m (3-quarter mile), 880m, 440m @ 10K race pace/moderately hard, with a 440m recovery
- Week 4—8 X 880m @10K race pace/moderately hard, with a 440m recovery
- Week 5—10 X 440m @ 5K race pace/hard, with a 220m recovery
- Week 6—3 X 1760m (1 mile) @ 10K race pace/moderately hard, with a 440m recovery
- Week 7—2 X 2 miles @ 10K race pace/moderately hard, with a 440m recovery
- Week 8—1 X 1760m, 1 X 2 mile, 1 X 1760m @ 10K pace/ moderately hard, with a 440m recovery
- Week 9—10 X 880m (half mile) @ 10K pace/moderately hard, with a 440m recovery, 5 minute rest after repeat number 5
- Week 10—4 X 1760m @ 10K race pace/moderately hard, with a 440m recovery

The Magical Year

By 1996, I had worked in the same office for eight years. I enjoyed working for the Labor Board and wanted to stay there, but I also wanted to do something different. So I became an appellate litigator for my agency, defending its decisions before the U.S. Courts of Appeal. The first time I stood up at the podium to argue a case was a nerve-racking moment. The courtroom seemed huge, and was subtly designed to impart an aura of importance to the proceedings, as well as intimidate all who entered. As I looked up at the three judges who would hear my case, my heart felt like it was about to rip through my body. And then I began to speak. "May it please the Court, my name is Jeff Horowitz, and I represent the National Labor Relations Board."

Suddenly, calmness came over me, and I felt completely at ease as I laid out the facts and the law for the judges, answering their questions and deflecting any criticism. It only lasted 10 minutes—average for an appellate argument—but when it was over, I felt an incredible sense of power and release. I loved it. Some attorneys in my office loved the grind of writing the briefs we had to submit, and dreaded oral argument, but I was the opposite. I liked the immediacy and danger of appearing in court.

It was almost as good as finishing a marathon. Almost. But compared to the adrenaline rush of the marathon finish line, it was no contest. Racing was my drug of choice.

Still, I had a lot to learn. In May, I flew to Cleveland for the old Revco Marathon. Having already run twenty-one marathons, I thought myself invincible, so I went out for Chinese food the night before the big race. Spicy eggplant. It turned on me at about mile 14 of the course the next day. Of course, there were no portable toilets anywhere in sight just then, and as I snuck down a dark alleyway, clutching the biggest leaves I could find, I swore that I would never take any chances again.

So, I was not invincible. Lesson learned.

Even with all my mistakes, I was still doing an awful lot right, and I had my breakthrough year in 1997. I had been doing speed work regularly, and was doing my long weekend runs with a fast bunch of guys. I felt quick and strong, and as the 1997 racing season, I felt an upsurge of confidence. I knew with great certainty that I would set a personal record every time I raced.

I was right. I ran a 5K in under 20 minutes, a 10-mile race in 62 minutes, and a half-marathon in 1:27. In late September, I ran marathon number 30 in East Lyme, Connecticut, in 3:12:57. Only 3 minutes separated me from the Boston Marathon. I began to believe it was possible.

I was scheduled to run my next marathon three weeks later in Detroit. It was a well-organized race with potential: a fast, flat course, not too big a field. I drove out there with my running buddies, who were also racing, and patiently waited for the race. We went to a University of Michigan football game, toured the city, ate, and rested. Finally, it was time to run.

The Detroit Marathon actually started in Canada, and boasted the only underground mile in marathoning, as runners were herded through a tunnel back to the United States. As with every marathon, the air seemed to crackle with energy as we waited for the race to start. My friends and I began as a pack, hoping to run together for as long as possible. As we ran, I happened to notice one woman in particular, running directly in front of me. My eyes traced down her long blond hair to her blue running tights, stretched taut over her lean body. Her stride was beautiful, and utterly mesmerizing. After a few seconds that seemed like an eternity, I sheepishly looked away. Glancing left and right, I saw that a row of five or six guys, including my friends, all had their eyes glued to the same spot. As if on cue, we all looked up, noticed each other, and broke into embarrassed laughter.

The early miles flew by. I separated from my friends and surged forward, settling into my target pace. As I moved into the second half of the race, I felt strong and was running well. I suddenly understood the pressure of having an ambitious time goal; every mile marker brought a quick recalculation of pace and split times. I counted down miles and counted seconds, and I knew that I had none to spare. In my previous thirty marathons, I was able to run relaxed, losing myself in the joy of the moment and in my thoughts, but not in Detroit. I spent precious energy trying to concentrate on the task at hand, to keep focused for mile after mile, hour after hour. It was excruciating. I used to daydream about being an elite runner, trading my desk for a schedule of full-time training and racing. It used to sound like heaven, but not any more; I realized that being a professional runner must be hard work.

With a mile to go, I was still on pace to qualify for Boston. I was tired and my muscles ached, but I knew that I only had minutes of pain left, and a lifetime to recover. *I could do this*, I thought. Being a marathoner meant that you were the kind of person who kept running when other people would quit. I was a marathoner. I would not quit. I pushed as hard as I could, my mind focused only on the rhythm of my running. Finally the finish line was in view. Flying across, I checked my time. 3:08:59. I had done it! A new personal best, and a qualifying time. I was going to return to Boston, and no one could say that I didn't deserve to be there.

But my big year wasn't over yet. I decided to risk mailing in an application for a race I wasn't sure I could even finish: the JFK 50 Mile. The name alone scared me. I had never before run an ultramarathon, and the thought of nearly doubling my longest race distance seemed insane. That, of course, is exactly what drew me to it. As intoxicating as it is to finish a marathon, something irretrievable is lost when that goal is first achieved: the fear that you cannot do it. The excitement that goes with that uncertainty is gone forever. After the finish line is crossed, the only question that remains for the future is whether you can do it again, or do it faster. Usually that's a good thing, but I found myself missing the unknown, missing the fear. When I mailed in my 50-miler race application, I felt a deep nervousness that I hadn't felt in years. After returning from Detroit, I gave myself a little recovery time, and then committed to myself to training with a fresh sense of urgency.

I did have several factors in my favor. First, I was already an accomplished marathoner, which meant that my body had become adept at relying on fat to fuel my running, instead of just glycogen. I had covered enough miles to make this adaptation, so I was confident that I would have an easier time transitioning to an ultramarathon than a beginning recreational runner would have transitioning to a regular marathon.

The second factor that calmed me was my realization that the longer the race distance, the less important it was to cover the target distance in training. This was reassuring; I wouldn't have to do a 50-mile training run in order to prepare for a 50-mile race. From everything I had read, the consensus seemed to be that a 35-mile run would give me a sufficient endurance base to conquer the JFK. Running 35 miles sounded much easier than running 50, which made this whole enterprise seem much more possible.

Still, 35 miles is still a long way to run by yourself. I would have to plan a way to get access to the supplies I would need. One option would be to just carry the food and drink I'd require, but that didn't sound too appealing, since I was looking at a 5-hour session. Another option would be to map out a route and stash food and drink on the course, but that didn't seem like a great idea either, since I couldn't be sure that the stuff I'd left out in plain view hours earlier would still be there when I really needed it. What I really needed, I thought, was to have refreshment stops, manned by volunteers, just like they have in the marathon. That's when the obvious solution hit me: I would use a full marathon as a training run, making full use of the course support throughout, and simply add another 9 miles of running at the end. Brilliant.

The race I chose was the Vulcan Marathon in Birmingham, Alabama, which was scheduled just three weeks after the Detroit Marathon, and just three weeks before the JFK. In addition to the perfect symmetry of this timetable, racing in Birmingham would add Alabama to the list of states I had run. I talked Dave into joining me—getting him to agree to run a marathon was like talking a kid into eating candy—and we flew down to Birmingham together.

Being from the Northeast, I thought sophistication ended at the Mason-Dixon line, but I discovered that Birmingham had beautiful neighborhoods, golf courses, and thriving shopping districts nestled within the city's boundaries. It was a good lesson to learn: there was a lot about this country that I knew nothing about.

On race day, Dave and I decided to abandon our all-out approach to marathoning, and instead committed ourselves to finishing the race together—no small accomplishment with pedal-to-the-metal Dave!—with a goal finish time of 3:30. I knew this meant that we'd both have to show restraint at different times, but as the race unfolded, I knew that we were doing the right thing. Not only was I reserving enough energy to continue running after I crossed the finish line, I was also enjoying having Dave as my companion throughout the race. Our shared racing goals had created a special bond, and the Vulcan Marathon seemed a fitting celebration of our brotherhood.

When the finish line came within view, we tried our best to cross the line at exactly the same time—3:31, within one minute of our goal. The official race Web site ended up awarding Dave the win by a few seconds, which led to endless ribbing. But that was later. After crossing the finish line, I still had work to do. I collected my medal and set out back on a street parallel to the course.

I was feeling surprisingly spry, and after running about 4.5 miles, I reversed course and dove back into the crowd of marathoners heading toward the finish line. It was a strange experience for me, since I was surrounded by runners who I never really got to see before: the back-of-the-pack runners who usually finished in 5 or 6 hours. As I weaved though them, I got more than one confused look from people who must have been wondering how I could be running so hard and still be so far back. I got more puzzled looks and comments from the aid station volunteers who recognized me from my first pass. I just shrugged and smiled and raced onward. When I got to the finish line, I veered off the course, and fought off the well-meaning and urgent directions of volunteers who tried to guide me into the finisher's chutes. I pulled out my medal and smiled. I had finished another marathon, but more importantly, I believed that I was ready for the JFK.

The JFK 50 Miler is legendary among ultramarathoners. It was inaugurated in 1963, after President Kennedy challenged his military staffers to complete a 50-mile hike in a single day. The race quickly grew into one of the largest ultramarathons in the country, with a starting field of 700–1,000 runners. That's a lot of crazy people in one place.

They would have to be fast, too; the JFK has a finishing cutoff time of 14 hours, with several checkpoints. Runners who failed to reach the checkpoints within the cutoff times would be removed from the course.

But for those who completed the race, there would be glory and bragging rights: according to the race Web site, less than one-tenth of 1 percent of Americans have completed a 50-mile race. Elite company indeed.

I thought about this as I lay down the night before the race. I kept thinking about the number 50. Suddenly, I just couldn't see any way that I could possibly finish the race. It was just too long. I'd been fooling myself; I'd never make it. Then I thought of something my mother had once told me: gambling is wrong, she said, but if I wanted to bet on something, I should bet on myself. Something clicked for me when I thought of that. I would take a chance on me. With that, I drifted off to sleep.

The JFK 50 Miler is held in Hagerstown, Maryland, conveniently located just a few hours from where I lived. On race day I woke up well before dawn and drove to the start, where I found a large group of mostly older, often heavier runners milling about at the local school, which served as the race day headquarters. It was a different sort of racing crowd than I expected. I thought everyone would look lean and sinewy, their bodies worn down to just the essentials. Instead, I saw some a lot of portly runners who looked to me like they might not even be able to make it around the block. We filed over to the race start in the darkness, and at the blast of the starter's gun we began our journey.

The race began on city streets, and as we ran, I eavesdropped on the conversations around me. These runners, even the heavier ones, talked about having run the JFK numerous times, and other ultras as well. These were experienced guys. At that moment I decided to stop judging them by their shape, and instead credit their accomplishments and try to follow their lead. When they began to walk on the upgrades, I followed suit, and when they paused at aid stations and ate the sandwiches and soup that were offered, I did that, too. This wouldn't guarantee me success, but it would put the odds in my favor.

The race soon led us onto the Appalachian Trail. I wasn't an experienced trail runner, but I thought that the trail portions chosen for the race would surely be the easiest available. Oh, was I wrong. The trail meandered up and down on rough, uneven paths, over rocks, boulders and exposed branches. I was soon acquainted with the agony of stubbed toes and sore ankles. I became so focused on my foot placement that I failed to see a thick, low-lying branch in my path. I ran smack into it headfirst. Everything flashed bright white, and I could hear a distant voice asking if I was okay. I mumbled "yes," and hoped it was true.

Eventually, we left the trail, and ran onto the C&O canal towpath. I was familiar with the canal from the portion of it that ends in D.C. While I had never been this far out on it, I knew that it would be a flat, hard-pack dirt path. We were to run 26 miles on it, almost a full marathon. I was already sore and tired, and doubted if I would be able to finish the race, but I was determined not to drop out unless things got much worse. They would have to pull me off the course for failing to hit the cutoff times. Otherwise, I'd keep moving forward.

The race became an exercise in myopia; I tried to forget how much road lay before me, and concentrated only on getting to the next mile marker, and the next aid station. At each station I swallowed down as much food as I could handle, and then shuffled forward. My pace dropped to little more than a fast walk, but I was not alone. Others around me were in the same condition, or worse. One runner was so disoriented that he failed to notice a hip-level barrier that we had to circle. He hit it full-stride and flipped over onto his back. Undeterred and uncomplaining, he slowly arose and resumed running, mechanically but relentlessly.

The mile markers came and went, conveying impossible-sounding information. Mile 30, mile 31, mile 32. At mile 35, a strange thing happened; I began to feel better. I stopped taking walk breaks, and picked up the pace. By the time I exited the canal for a final 8 miles on the roads, I had sped up to a respectable 8:30-per-mile pace. Darkness descended as I raced those final miles, and when the finish line loomed before me, in front of a local high school, I looked up at the clock and smiled in disbelief. Nine hours 24 minutes. I had run all day, from predawn to nightfall. Even as I collected my medal, I couldn't believe I had done it. There was still the long drive home, though, and the fact of my race set in firmly as my legs ached and my muscles sagged. I had never felt so tired and sore, not even after my very first marathon. I would need weeks to fully recover physically, and almost as long to recover my desire to race.

So what to make of this? What was I to do with an ultramarathon finish? Could I add it to my list of marathons? After all, it was *at least* a marathon. That seemed fair enough. But even as I wrote it down, I knew it couldn't stay on the list. I was committed to running marathons, and that's a precise distance. I was free to run any other distance also, but they could not be included on the list. I could not add four 10Ks together and call them a marathon, and neither could I divide my marathons into eight separate 5K-plus finishes. My totals would be precise and beyond question; I had officially run thirty-two marathons and one *ultra*marathon.

The JFK 50 brought an end to my 1997 racing campaign. There were still adventures to be had in my future, exotic journeys and great races, but there would never again be a year for me quite like 1997.

Running Tip #3

Form Drills

Drills break down the running motion into distinct movements and improve running efficiency, form, and speed. Once a week, find a 50-meter stretch of road or track. Warm up and do each of these drills 2–4 times, taking a 30-second recovery between each repeat.

- *Butt kicks.* Take short steps while kicking your heels up as high as you can. This drill strengthens the hamstrings, a primary muscle group used in running.
- *High steps.* Take short steps as you pick your knees up as high as they can go. This drill strengthens the calves and hip flexors, which is the area where the bottom of your abdomen meets your leg—a muscle group that's crucial to the running motion, and emphasizes proper running posture and the lift-off phase of running.
- *High Skips.* Swing your arms strongly and skip as high as you can. This drill helps build explosive power in your running stride to improve hill-running and a strong finishing kick in your racing.
- *Stiff-legged Running.* Also called "soccer kicks." Run on your toes, keeping your legs locked out as straight as possible the entire time. This drill will also strengthen the hip flexors.
- *Strides.* Don't sprint; run hard but in control, with an emphasis on monitoring your form. This drill gives you a chance to work on any inefficiency in your form, and prepares your body for the next phase of your workout—your actual distance run—by lengthening your stride.

Pain, Fear, and Faith

As my marathon total climbed, I found that people weren't asking me why I ran out of admiration now so much as with concern. Many of them had seemed to become suspicious about my running. They began calling me obsessed, in that "I'm joking but you should really think about this" kind of way, and seemed to assume that my running enabled me to avoid dealing with some deeper, darker issues. They said that I must be running away from something.

I didn't think that was true. Running wasn't an escape; if anything, it was a lantern in the dark, a mirror showing me things about myself that I had to face. I could no sooner run away from my problems than I could run away from my own body; when I ran, there was only the road, my thoughts, and time. Eventually, inevitably, I would have to think about anything troubling me. Perhaps it was the rhythm of my footsteps that calmed me down and sharpened my thinking, or perhaps I just reacted well to the rush of endorphins, but whatever the reason, when I ran I saw things more clearly, and could see answers to questions that seemed insolvable only hours before.

Do you remember that poem, "Footprints in the Sand"? Sure you do. You've seen it on automobile air fresheners and on cheesy plaques at every truck stop you've ever wandered into. It goes like this: A man looked back on the path he'd traveled all his life and saw that although the Lord often walked by his side, during the most difficult times, there was only one set of footprints in the sand. The man turned to the Lord and asked, "Why did you abandon me when I needed you the most?" The Lord answered, "Oh, my son, it was then that I carried you."

I hate that story. Not just because it's the worst kind of corny, dime-store religious palaver, although that's exactly what it is; I hate it because it turns me to mush. Every time I read it, my heart rises into my throat and my eyes begin to moisten. Good god, that's actually happening to me right now. I just can't help it, and it's infuriating.

My running reminds me of that story. During the hardest times of my life—when I lost loved ones, when my heart was broken, when I was studying for the bar exam, and whenever I felt alone in the world—running was there for me, providing some relief from my troubles, putting things in perspective and letting me see that the road always continued onward. My running carried me and sustained me.

I've always thought that everyone should have some activity in their lives in which they can become so immersed that they lose track of time. When that happens, when there is no past or future, but only the present, you can find a little bit of that most rare commodity: a little peace of mind. When I relax on a long run, I can get to that place, and in that relaxed state, I can see answers to the problems in my life, and put things in perspective.

This is especially true on my longest runs. During a shorter run of six to eight miles, I know that I'll be finished within an hour, give or take a few minutes. That run becomes a small part of the day's plan, and during the run, I find myself looking ahead to what I need to take care of next when the workout is over, and sometimes I get impatient to be finished so I can get on with the day's chores. But on an 18- to 20-mile run, I know that I'll be on the road for hours, and when I'm finished, I'll be in no mood to rush off to tackle other projects and run errands. The long run becomes the 500-pound gorilla sitting in the middle of a room, completely impossible to ignore. On those days, I give in to the gorilla, and settle into a comfortable pace, knowing that there is nothing else that I need to concern myself with other than putting one foot in front of the other. Any impatience that I might have had during shorter runs disappears. On the long days, there's just me, the road, and endless time.

Not that running is always a pleasure. Running, especially marathon racing, also brings pain. During the last miles of a marathon, my quadriceps muscles are often aching, my hamstrings might be complaining, my calves are possibly cramping, and even my shoulders are fatigued. None of this surprises me; in fact, all of it is entirely expected. I think of these aches and pains as old friends come to visit. I even welcome them, since they signal to me that I'm back in familiar territory, and that the end of the race must be near.

I don't usually talk about these aches and pains with nonrunners, though, because I don't think they'll understand. It's not that marathon runners are masochists—at least not in the traditional sense, and certainly not most of them. It's just that pain means something else to us than it means to most other people. To a runner, pain is a sign of achievement; it's proof that we've expended the maximum effort. When our sides ache from oxygen debt and our legs burn with lactic acid build-up, or when we spend the days after a hard race hobbling pitifully up and down stairs, we know that we had run as hard as we possibly could. The pain, then, is not a cause for concern; it's a cause for celebration. And when we feel perfectly fine after finishing a race, we hear a little voice inside asking us whether it might be true that we could have run faster than we did. In fact, one of my running fantasies is to collapse immediately after finishing a marathon, having used my very last measure of energy to throw myself across the finish line for a new personal best. That would be a perfect race.

But I don't actually enjoy the pain. It's not fun to cool down after a race and discover that your body has stiffened up so much that you could no longer easily or painlessly step down from the curb to the street. Nor is there easy rest for a weary body when every toss and turn in the middle of the night brings complaints from sore muscles, and every attempt to stand up from a chair takes minutes rather than seconds. This kind of pain is humbling; it's disruptive not only to a regular workout routine, but to any kind of normal life. It's a deep-to-the-bone kind of soreness that I would never have known if I had never run a marathon.

The memory of these aches leads me to look down at my legs with pity at every starting line, since they don't know yet what hell I'm about to put them through. But after an hour or two of running, they'll figure it out, and brace themselves for the familiar challenge. If they could speak, perhaps they would tell me not to worry. They understand that this pain is fleeting; we have weathered it before, and we can weather it again. Just get on with it, they would say.

Actual injuries are an entirely different story. There is no long-time runner who hasn't experienced their share of sprains, strains, fractures, and tears. Get a group of runners together, and before long they'll start talking about their injury histories, like war veterans comparing battle scars. During those moments, it might be easy to believe that runners don't mind being injured, but that's dead wrong. If the storytellers are smiling, it's only because the injuries are healed, or because they're trying not to let their frustration show. Dealing with an injury is often a greater test of a runner's resolve than any grueling workout or race.

Once I began to run marathons on a regular basis, many of my friends predicted that my bones would turn to dust, and I'd be crippled within just a few years. Some doctors said much the same thing.

The injuries that I sometimes struggled with only seemed to confirm their predictions. After overcoming that bad ankle sprain in 1986, I suffered a sequence of regular setbacks over the next few years. At one point I had terrible back spasms and had to undergo physical therapy, and another time I developed pain in my knees due to tightness in the muscle and connective tissue that runs along the outside of our legs, called the ilio-tibial band. On a less serious but no less painful side, I also developed awful-looking blisters during my early races. I tried to prevent them by slathering my feet with petroleum jelly, or wrapping each toe with medical tape. In desperation, I once both wrapped and jellied my feet. Not a good idea. By race's end, I was left with a slippery mass of balled up tape jammed in the front of my shoes.

Another time, I felt a blister developing on my right pinky toe early in a race. Being an old pro by this point, I pulled over to an aid station and wrapped tape around the toe. Problem solved. I jumped back in the race and ran smoothly for the next 19 miles, but after crossing the 26 mile marker, with the finish line within sight just up ahead, I suddenly felt a very painful pop in my right foot. I was quickly reduced to a hobble, and I was sure that I had torn a ligament in that pinky toe. After pulling myself across the finish line, I staggered straight to the medical tent, where I sat down and pulled of my right shoe. The end of my sock was covered in blood. I pulled off the sock, and then had a medical technician carefully cut the tape along the length of my toe. I slowly pulled the tape back, and gazed at what I saw underneath. The toe was a raw stick of meat. Stuck on the tape was my skin and toenail. Slowly, it dawned on me what had happened. I had developed a blister underneath the toenail, and finally, at mile 26, it popped violently, unhinging both the nail and the surrounding skin. Luckily, it didn't feel as bad as it looked, but whenever I want to make someone cringe, I pull that story out from my bag of tales.

Eventually, I found the right combination of treatments to get my feet safely through my races, and eventually they seemed to just toughen up and blister less frequently. My other injuries also healed and disappeared, leaving me wiser. I began to see my body as a kind of minefield which I could traverse only by stepping carefully around the spots where I knew explosives lay. *Not there! You'll get a sore knee if you do that. And that will hurt your back!*

Despite all of those training and racing woes, however, I came to realize over the years that I was actually a very durable runner. I had a stable stride an unusually large vastus medialis—the muscle above the kneecap that helps hold the kneecap in place. Like most other runners, I still had to work on my flexibility and strengthen the muscles in my back and abdominal areas, but I had come to realize that while I might not be the fastest runner in the field, I was built to keep running.

Still, if I have a different relationship to pain than most nonrunners, I also have a different collection of fears. Preparing for and running the JFK 50 Mile led me to consider again the role of fear in running, since, for the first time in a very long while, I had ventured outside of my comfort zone into unknown territory. By that time I was very confident that I could run a marathon. After all, I had already run thirty-two of them. But I was very worried about the JFK 50. I felt a fear of failure that I had not felt in years. It was a feeling that was unsettling and disturbing, though not entirely unpleasant.

Fear, like any stress, is a double-edged sword. Unhealthy and paralyzing in large doses, it's also essential for achievement, and leads to the cathartic hormonal release that we all find so pleasurable. This is the fear that we seek out and pay for with every horror movie and roller-coaster ride we experience. But runners live with a more common brand of fear, cousin more to insecurity than to terror. This is the fear that whispers in our ear that past achievement matters little because our bodies are no longer in the condition they were in a few months or even weeks ago. This is the fear that gains traction with every disappointing workout and slow training run we endure. It is the fear that undermines our confidence day by day, replacing it with gnawing doubt.

Runners, like many other people, seek to conquer our fears by clinging to ritual. We have our lucky socks and hats, our favorite old shirts and shoes. We swear by our food choices, our race-morning routines, and our prerace warm-up. Some of these rituals are rooted in experimentation that would make a scientist proud, while others are shrouded in superstition and faith. For example, I personally would never wear a race's shirt before finishing that race. It's a *finisher's* shirt, after all, and wearing it before you cross the finish line could result in a powerful jinx. It just makes sense. Or, at least, it does to me. But however established, these rituals and superstitions hang on with the tenacity of a pit bull, because to a runner, preparation is everything, and if we repeat the exact details that led to past success, then that success can be replicated. We convince ourselves that there will be no failure, no shame, no heartbreak on this day, because we have done everything right. With all the necessaries attended to, success should follow, as surely as night follows day. Fear is conquered.

In a larger sense, though, our fear is not about a single training session, or a particular race. It is about our mortality; it is about our knowledge that there is a limit to our improvement. We know that eventually, inevitably, age, the swiftest runner, will catch us and hang on our backs. Our legs will slow, our finishing times will climb like the temperature on a sweltering day, and we'll realize that we're one mile closer to the end of our life's race. We run every workout and race under this cloud. Just as running fulfills the promise of life, it contains within it the seeds of decline.

But we need not give into this fear. With every strong workout, every fast lap, every personal best, we push the darkness back. To do so requires determination, and yes, pain. Speed workouts hurt, racing hard hurts, but we do it. We do it to push away the fear, to hold onto the illusion of immortality one more moment. To live fully, completely.

With experience, we can learn not to despair with every slow run, secure in the knowledge that a great workout will likely soon follow. Even an occasional bad race won't be the harbinger of doom. Eventually, we know, decline will set in. But not today, not here, not now. I will muzzle this fear, and cover the Earth in great hungry strides, cheating time and decay with every step for as long as I can.

As I pondered these thoughts, I began to see the human body as something of a divine instrument, and running itself as an expression of faith and an affirmation of the wonder of life. This was my private belief, though, and I wasn't eager to make a public declaration of it. Religion was, I felt, a private matter, and I wasn't interested in expressing my views to anyone who might not be interested in hearing about them.

Not everyone else agreed. I once heard about Catherine Ndereba, the great four-time Boston Marathon champion and 2004 Olympic silver medalist, when she graciously spoke to a small crowd of runners before the Barbados Marathon in 2003. She was open and warm, and everything you could hope for in a celebrity.

But Catherine began her talk by thanking God for her accomplishments, and referred again and again to her faith as the source of her power. I shifted uneasily, and I thought I saw others do the same. We weren't interested in talking about religion; we wanted to talk about running, and questions from the crowd steered her away from religion by asking her instead about her training schedule and her views on her competitors. I respect Catherine's beliefs, and admire her great ability, determination, and courage, but I didn't much like being preached to.

I came to feel uncomfortable with another expression of faith in the running community as well: those runners who literally wear their beliefs of their sleeves. I began seeing slogans like "With God All Things Are Possible" splashed across their shirts, followed in short order by others bearing biblical quotes and psalms. Not what I would do, but it really wasn't any of my business. But then one day I passed a runner with a shirt declaring "Jesus is my coach." Really? What speed work does Jesus recommend for marathoners? Does Jesus believe in effort-based training, or does He use a stopwatch? Does Jesus recommend supplements? Of course, I said none of those things to him; I didn't want be rude or offensive. But flip declarations of faith are, in my view, little more than advertising slogans, and I don't like them.

There is a role for faith in running, as in all of life. All runners have faith, of one kind or another; it's what enables us to try going beyond the limits that we once thought would stop us. But all runners know, too, that faith is only the safety net; real achievement comes from our own sweat, from our conscious choice to sacrifice and work hard. Making choices is the foundation for all morality, and rather than relying on faith to guide us in our actions, we should fashion our actions to reflect our faith. Running, to me, is what the cathedral was to the masses in the Middle Ages: a visible declaration of the wonder of creation. For me, running is the best expression of a runner's faith. Through pain and injury, and success, we are who we are, and become who we want to be.

My quest continued.

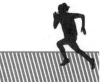

Running Tip #4

Dealing with Injuries

Injuries happen. The trick is not just to avoid injury, but to respond intelligently when you feel one coming on. If you respond quickly and correctly when you develop a problem, you'll be back running at 100 percent in almost no time at all. Generally, cutting back on training, and stretching, strengthening, and icing the area will help. Thinking that you could just bully your body into submission, however, will *not* work. Trust me, I know.

Here's a short list of the most common training ailments, with suggested treatments. As with any injury, if symptoms persist for more than a week or two, worsen, or if the pain feels sharp rather than dull, you should see a doctor.

- *Black toe.* The toenail turns black, and sometimes falls off. This is a sign that your shoes are too small, and the toe is jamming against the front of the shoe, resulting in bruising of the nail bed. The fix? Buy shoes that are at least a half size or more larger than your dress shoes.
- *Knee pain—on the front.* This is probably patella tendonitis, and is caused by excessive movement of the knee cap over the knee joint. Insufficient muscle strength in the front of the upper leg—the quadriceps muscles, particularly on the inner side—is usually to blame. Do leg strengthening exercises such as squats, leg presses, or lunges.

→

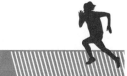

- *Knee pain—on the outside.* Called iliotibial band syndrome, this is an inflammation of the muscle and connective tissue running from the upper front hip bone (ilium) down along the outside of the leg, over the outside of the knee, down to the kneecap and calf (tibia bone). Tightness causes the IT band to rub against the outside of the knee, causing pain. Treat with ice and self-massage, and stretch until you feel tightness in your hip and backside.
- *Knee pain—on the back of the knee.* This is often caused by tightness in the hamstrings. Stretch your hamstrings and do self-massage.
- *Pain on the heel or arch.* This is likely plantar fasciitis, an inflammation of the connective tissue in that area. A common indicator of plantar fasciitis is pain in the arch first thing in the morning. Treat with gentle stretching and icing.
- *Pain on the front of the lower leg/shin.* Likely shin splints, a result of training too intensely too soon, especially on hard surfaces. Ice by massaging the area with a frozen cup of water, holding the open end on the affected area. Strengthen the area by doing "duckwalks"—walking once a day back and forth across a room on your heels with your toes up in the air for 5–10 minutes.

Mountain Madness

In the summer of 1998, I was just over a third of the way to my 100-marathon goal—close enough to claim to know what I was doing, but far enough to still not be able to imagine actually achieving it. When I sat down and thought about all the miles and races before me, I felt farther away from my goal than ever. I realized that the only way to keep on my path was to ignore that I was on it; by refusing to acknowledge how far I had to go, I would be able to keep putting one foot in front of the other. It was the same strategy that I used in each race I ran. As I told people, I never imagined running 26.2 miles at a time—I saw myself as running a single mile twenty-six times in a row. Somehow, it that made all the difference. But now, to reach the ultimate finish line, I would have to extend this trick to years, not just hours.

Some runners seem to maintain their motivation through familiarity, returning to the same races year after year, like salmon returning to their spawning grounds. They find comfort in running familiar ground, and take pride in not missing a single edition of their favorite races. Or perhaps they discover new, subtle things about the course every time they run them, like a Shakespearean scholar who finds new meaning and artistry with every reading of *Macbeth*.

That's not me. I have run certain marathons multiple times—Boston, New York, and the Marine Corps Marathon—but by and large I want to see something new and different every time I race. For me, there's no greater way to experience a new place than on the run, and there's no better way to distract myself from pain and fatigue than by running down unfamiliar roads. That's really why I began to travel to run in the first place.

Of course, not all races are created equal; some are more exotic and challenging than others. And then there are some that some races that are so far off the beaten path that it seems misleading to simply call them marathons. The Pikes Peak Marathon is one such race.

Pikes Peak is a 14,110-foot-high granite mountain in central Colorado, thrusting skyward from the city of Colorado Springs, with the smaller town of Manitou Springs hugging its eastern flank. The fledgling United States gained title over the mountain in the Louisiana Purchase, and it was named for Zebulon Pike, the man President Jefferson sent to survey the southwestern border of the new territory in 1806. Pike tried to scale the mountain, but was turned back by a blizzard. The summit was finally conquered in 1820, but the surrounding area wasn't settled for another fifty years. In 1873, the U.S. Army built a weather station on the summit, and by 1888 a toll road had been built to the top. A cog railroad was soon added, and by 1901 the first automobile climbed the peak. In 1918, a hiking trail to the top was completed, named the Barr Trail, for the father and son team who constructed it.

Once it became possible to reach the top, human nature being what it is, people began to challenge each other to race to the summit. An auto race was held in 1916, and then, on Sunday, June 28, 1936, twenty-five men and two women lined up for the first Pikes Peak footrace. Nineteen made it to the top. Twenty years would pass before another such race was attempted.

On Friday, August 10, 1956, fourteen runners lined up to race once more to the top, this time in honor of the 150th anniversary of Zebulon Pike's mission. According to legend, the race was the result of a bet between smokers and nonsmokers. As it turned out, no one fared especially well, as only four people made it to the summit. But the race had touched something in people's imagination, and this time it would not die. It was held again the following year, and then again, until it became an established event. Slowly the field of participants grew from a handful of lunatics the first several years, to several hundred lunatics by the 1970s, and then to several thousand lunatics by the 1990s. It turned out that there was a bottomless supply of lunatics who wanted to throw themselves at the mountain, but because the Barr Trail was too narrow to allow a large field of runners, most of these would-be ascenders had to be turned away. Despite the difficulty of getting into the race, or perhaps because of it, enthusiasm for the event grew. The Pikes Peak Marathon had become an institution.

I wasn't aware of any of this history in 1998 when I mailed off my application to Colorado. I just wanted this race to be my thirty-seventh marathon. Lady Luck must have smiled on my application, though, because soon I received a confirmation of entry, along with a twenty-page information booklet. I was a bit mystified. Usually prerace instructions aren't longer than a page or two. But this booklet had twenty pages of instructions and warnings. *Twenty pages!* What had I gotten myself into?

I kicked off my shoes, threw myself onto my couch, and began to read. What surprised me about the race was the sheer volume of things to worry about. First, of course, was the climb. While most marathons have a significant hill or two, this one was nothing *but* hill; runners climb 7,815 feet up, and then race 7,815 feet down. The toll on the legs would be staggering, as muscles and joints would be tested in every possible way.

But that's not even the worst of it. The race *starts* at 6,295 feet above sea level, and climbs above the timberline where no tree can grow, into the thin air above 14,000 feet. At those heights, breathing becomes difficult, and running becomes almost unthinkable. The booklet recommended that participants train themselves in the technique of forced breathing, in which the diaphragm is repeatedly pushed to take in more air without exhausting the chest wall muscles.

But that wasn't even the worst of it. Apart from the climb and the altitude, there was the volatility of the summer weather on Pikes Peak to worry about. It was said to be utterly and dangerously unpredictable. "Pikes Peak can have rapid and extreme weather changes several times each day," the booklet warned. "Chilling rain, snow and sleet showers, high winds and dramatic temperature changes can occur [on race day] in August." The temperatures could drop by as much as fifty degrees from the starting line in Manitou Springs to the mountain peak. But that wasn't the real problem, the booklet insisted. The greatest danger to runners actually comes from sudden lightning storms above the tree line.

I put the booklet down and looked at the ceiling, pondering what I had just read. The contents of the booklet sounded frightening, and the chances for a flawless marathon looked slim. In fact, from the look of things, I would be lucky just to make it back alive and in one piece.

I smiled.

After conquering the challenge of simply getting into the race, I had to decide how to adjust my training to handle the unusual demands that the race would make on my body. The race organizers suggested arriving in Colorado two weeks before the event in order to begin acclimatizing to the altitude. Much as I would like to have done that, my boss, Uncle Sam, seemed to have other priorities, and I just couldn't take the time off. Other than constructing a hyperbaric tent over my bed to mimic high altitude—which I did consider for a hot second—my plan was just to fly out there the day before the race and hope for the best.

Training for the climb itself was also a matter of hope. I spent long hours laboring on the stepper machine and running hills, betting that would prepare me for the mountain. As for the dealing with the weather, I planned to bring enough gear to be prepared for any contingency. I packed layers and throwaway clothes—enough, really, for a week's worth of racing.

Finally, there was nothing left to do but rest and fly out to Colorado. I arrived in Manitou Springs in the early afternoon the day before the race, and spent some time walking around town before picking up my race packet. On the outskirts of town was the beautiful and aptly named Garden of the Gods, where a walking path snaked around pale red monoliths and rock outcrops. Manitou Springs itself looks like it had gracefully made the transition from mining town to tourist attraction, but without being infected with too much gaudiness. The streets were lined with small shops and restaurants nestled in century-old buildings. You had the feeling it wouldn't be all that unnatural to see a stagecoach rumble past. All this was interesting enough, but my thoughts were elsewhere. I wanted to get my race number and focus on the task at hand.

Usually, race organizers set up shop in a conference room of the host hotel, which is where you expect to go to pick up your race packet. Not so at Pikes Peak. Organizers set up their tables in a park, giving would-be racers a chance to look up at the Peak before they accepted their race number. Rather than filling runners with dread, however, the sight of the Peak seemed to inspire excitement in the race crowd. Newcomers and veterans alike seemed like so many greyhounds in the slip, waiting for the bell to ring. I tried to ignore it. I wanted to be calm, and save all my energy for the race.

The following morning I found myself shoulder to shoulder with other runners in Manitou Springs, near the park I had visited the day before. It was a cool morning, and I could see the breath of the runners around me as they stretched, pawed at the ground with their feet, and looked skyward toward our goal. This is the most difficult time for a runner—the twilight between preparing for a race and actually running.

There is nothing left to do but worry about things that had gone wrong in training, and there is not yet the reassurance that comes with actual racing, when the body tells you that everything will be okay. This is just the waiting, and it can seem endless.

That time passed, though, as it always does, and the blast of the starter's gun released us. We raced through town, past the storefronts and homes, seeking out the entrance to the Barr Trail. Soon we found it. We plunged into the woods and started to climb in earnest. Runners jockeyed for position on the narrow trail, eager to spend their nervous energy. I held my position, but I didn't worry too much about skipping ahead. Passing people was not going to be my concern this day; I just wanted to make it up and back in one piece.

The air was clean and fresh, and the leaves around me were a vivid green as I settled into a smooth rhythm. The climbs were mixed with flat stretches, where our footfalls were muffled by soft dirt. Eventually, I realized that the forest was thinning, and that the soaring trees were shrinking. Soon, they gave way to large bushes, and then they, too, disappeared, replaced by pale yellow and orange rock. We had reached the tree line, the point at which the forest had to turn back from the altitude and climate of the mountain. Now things would get interesting.

The sun shone brightly now as I made my way up the rocky incline. The gentleness of the forest floor had disappeared with the trees, and now I had to make my way over loose rock and sharp boulders. Looking up the distant cliff-side in front of me, I could see a line of tiny runners zigzagging the switchbacks, looking like ants on a foraging mission. To my left stretched out the vastness of the southwest and an endless blue sky. It was a beautiful sight, but like the siren's call, it could lead me to disaster if gazing at it caused me to stumble and fall on the rocks underfoot. This was not the time for long, admiring gazes toward distant peaks.

I came across Barr Camp, a little oasis on the trail where volunteers waited with water and snacks. Their enthusiasm was infectious, and I threw myself back on the trail with renewed energy. Soon, though, my breathing became labored, and I realized that it wasn't caused just by the steady climb; the air was getting thinner. Everyone around me was moving slowly, and I joined them in walking the steepest sections of trail. My head started throbbing, and I leaned back on a boulder to rest. I tried to breathe down into my stomach, drawing as much precious air into my lungs as possible. From my rocky perch, I could see runners dotting the trail below me, forming a jagged seam on the mountainside. Wisps of clouds appeared overhead, and I wondered what the temperature was at the peak. I recalled that the race materials said that the typical time up to the half-way point at the top was the same as an entire flatland marathon, plus one half hour. I was starting to believe it.

I took another deep breath and pushed myself off the rock, reclaiming a spot in the line of runners inching their way to the top. I looked up, trying to gauge how much more there was to climb, but every spot I had been sure was the top instead turned out to be only a bend in the trail. I knew I was getting close, though, because the lead runners passed me on their way back down. I marveled at how fresh they looked; while I was struggling to walk, they flew downhill. I couldn't imagine having that kind of energy. For that matter, I could hardly imagine running the 13 miles back down to the finish line, but I refused to let myself think about that. I concentrated on simply putting one foot in front of the other, and blocked out all other thoughts.

The air became cooler, but there weren't any of the dramatic weather changes that we had been warned about. I moved mechanically, gulping air, wondering if there was actually a top to this mountain. And then suddenly, there it was. I had made it up to 14,110 feet, the top floor. There was a visitor center at the top, and plenty of spectators to cheer us on, but there was no time to celebrate. The top of the trail led us through a narrow defile through the rock, where volunteers unceremoniously spun us around and pointed us back downhill.

I pivoted and began to move forward, and then discovered an amazing thing: I could run! And more than that, I could run fast. It was as if I was being sucked into a vortex, and I felt better with every step. I slid on the gravel and hopped over rocks and boulders, spinning on the switchbacks like a car burning rubber on a wild turn. I couldn't believe how great I felt. It was nothing short of miraculous.

I had read that the difference between suffering altitude sickness and feeling fine can be as little as several dozen feet. I don't know if that's true, but I can tell you that each step down restored my strength and confidence. I was having fun. I ate up great chunks of trail with each stride, offering encouragement to the runners still moving toward the top. Like watching a movie in reverse, I saw the bits of brush appear between the orange and yellow rock, followed by small bushes and stunted trees. Soon, I was back in the woods again, below the tree line.

I was still flying, but my legs had started to protest. As much fun as downhill running can be, it's still hell on the quads, which have to work overtime to keep their fool owner from toppling forward and doing a face-plant. Not a problem, though: I had learned long ago how to ignore my screaming legs. I was more concerned about the footing. Downhill running on trail and broken rock is usually a recipe for disaster, but so far I had no problem handling the challenge.

No sooner had that thought entered my mind, hanging in the air like a thought balloon in a comic strip, than I found myself sprawled on the ground with my ankle screaming in pain. I pulled myself upright and took a tentative step. More screaming from below. I had twisted my ankle badly, that much was obvious. But standing alone in the woods, with runners off in the distance in front and behind me, and help—in the form of a rest stop—miles farther down the road, I had no choice but to keep moving. I took a few more easy steps. Not as bad as I first thought, really, once I got moving. I tried an easy jog. That seemed manageable. As I continued running, the pain subsided. Perhaps the adrenaline coursing through my body had blocked it out, or perhaps my body had responded by releasing a good dose of cortisol, a natural anti-inflammatory. Whatever it was, I was grateful for it, and promised to reward my body with a stop at the next aid station to have my ankle wrapped.

With the toughest part of the course behind me, I knew I wouldn't drop out unless I had no choice. I quickly constructed a cost-benefit test: how much of a layoff would I be willing to accept to complete the race? A week? Certainly. A month? Sure. Several months. Well … I guess so. Permanent injury? No, of course not. But how could I tell which of these fates lay in my future if I kept running?

I decided to turn the question around: rather than worry about what might happen, I would look only for clues as to what would certainly happen. Unless permanent injury became obviously inevitable, I would keep running for as long as I could. At the next aid station a volunteer wrapped my ankle tightly, and I was off again, rolling downhill, betting on my ankle against the mountain.

The miles flew by, and soon I was reached the end of the trail. After so many hours of running on dirt and rock, it was strange to be on asphalt again. From there I only had a short piece of running through town to the finish line, and it was mostly downhill. Usually that would be welcome relief, but not now. My quads were screaming at me, and my toes jammed painfully into the front of my shoes with each step. I groaned out loud and rolled my eyes in agony; I didn't think I could stand much more. Finally, there was only one more corner to turn, and there it was: the finish line. The clock read 6 hours 58 minutes.

I collected my medal and sat down in a folding chair in the tent just past the finish line. I had been tested, but I had not broken. My ankle would recover, my toes would heal, and my legs would eventually forgive me, but this moment would never be forgotten.

Looking around me, though, I saw that my injuries paled in comparison to those sustained by other runners. The tent looked like an army triage center. There were bloody elbows and knees, as well as cut and bruised faces. There had obviously been a lot of falling up on the mountain. Despite all the blood and bruises, though, I didn't see any sad faces. We had all survived, and better still, had triumphed. The bloody bandage became a badge of honor, a sign of how close to the edge each of us had pushed ourselves.

Later that night, I laid my still-wrapped ankle on a pillow and slung a bag of ice over it. It was classic RICE therapy: Rest, Ice, Compression, and Elevation. I knew that was the proper way to treat a sprain, and I thought just this once I would play it by the book. I didn't have high expectations.

The next morning, I was surprised to find that the swelling of my ankle had gone down, and that the pain was mostly gone as well. This RICE thing actually worked. Who woulda thunk it? I was back running within just a few days, good as new. Better than new, actually, because I had conquered Pikes Peak, America's toughest marathon. I felt that victory in my 100-marathon quest was now assured. But if I thought that there would be no more challenges, I was greatly mistaken, as I would soon find out.

Running Tip #5

Race Recovery

- *Eat something 15–30 minutes after training or racing.* This will kick-start refueling of your muscles and repair of any cellular damage.
- *Take a cold bath, massage your legs, grab some couch time.* All of these will help move blood and waste products out of your legs.
- *Take the long view.* Plan on needing one day of rest or easy training for every hard mile you raced.
- *Get back to it slowly.* Run no longer than an hour at a time for the first few weeks after a hard marathon.
- *Beware the sniffles.* Your immune system takes a battering on race day, so get plenty of sleep, drink lots of fluids, eat well, wash your hands frequently, and avoid touching your eyes and nose.

Why Run the Marathon? Second Lap

The question would not go away. I would go days and weeks without thinking about it, but sooner or later I would figuratively reach into my pocket, pull it out, sit it on a table, and look at it. Why run the marathon? I couldn't seem to find a good, complete answer to that question.

In the years following my first marathon, I had pursued my growing passion for fitness and became a certified personal trainer and running coach, filling my early morning and evening hours with sessions in a local gym, and my weekends coaching charity fund-raising marathon teams. I became a fitness evangelist, preaching and living the healthy life. I did not want to induce any delusions of immortality, though. I told my clients at our first session that our goal was to improve where we could, maintain as best we're able, and extend the quality of our life; nothing less, but nothing more.

This sounded right to me, but it opened a door onto bigger questions. I thought about something I once read former New York Mets and Philadelphia Phillies relief pitcher Tug McGraw had said. After blowing a game, he would ponder something he called the Ice Ball Theory, which went something like this: some day, many millions of years from now, our sun will become a supernova, scorch the earth, and then flame out into nothingness. After that, our planet will wander eternity in a dark void, a giant ice ball hurtling through space. At that point, no one will be around to care that on a sunny afternoon Tug McGraw once served up a home run pitch to lose a baseball game. Tug found it much easier to sleep at night after running that scenario through his mind.

The problem with the Ice Ball Theory, as I soon realized, was that it proved too much. Instead of just showing how little any one mistake matters in the scheme of things, it showed how *nothing* really matters. Not a very comforting idea after all. The question for me, then, became not just why run the marathon, but instead, if all achievement and failure eventually fade into the void equally, why bother doing anything at all?

These philosophical musings suddenly took on an unexpected urgency. One of my new clients, Burt, told me that he was HIV positive, and that he was also undergoing chemotherapy. He seemed uncomfortable talking about his health, and I didn't press for details beyond what I needed to know as his trainer, but I did tell him that I was proud of him for taking control of his life and for trying to improve himself. It was the type of life-affirming act that brought me into training in the first place.

Burt had more body fat than he should have been carrying, and he wasn't as strong as he wanted to be. His self-esteem had also taken a battering from the disease. I knew that training him would be a challenge for both of us. We began slowly, getting him comfortable with the exercises, discovering his limits, and gently pushing them to new levels. As time went by, Burt was amazed to see his strength improving. Soon, he told me, his friends noticed as well, and commented on his changed appearance. Burt also experienced a change of attitude: instead of being the victim of his disease, he began to show confidence and a new enthusiasm for life. I was accustomed to helping people get results, but this was something new for me. Something special was happening.

One day I called Burt to set up another appointment. He sounded scared and very upset. He was feeling very ill, and he told me that a friend was about to take him to the hospital. I told him not to jump to any conclusions, since he had been feeling so good for so long. We would just keep an open mind and wait to hear what the doctors had to say. He promised to call me as soon as he felt up to it.

I was very busy at the time, and several weeks passed before I realized how long it had been since I'd spoken with him. I was filled with dread as I punched his phone number, made infinitely worse when I was patched through into another employee's voice mail. I left several messages at his home number that I hoped sounded calm and upbeat, but that urged him to call me.

Finally he called. It turned out that he had had a bad reaction to the various medications that he was taking. His doctors had given him a transfusion and kept him in the hospital for a week. He had lost a lot of weight and strength, but what was worse, he had also lost his confidence and sense of purpose, and was depressed about the big step backward that he had taken in his fitness program. He said that he doubted that he could get back to where he was before his illness. Not to worry, I told him. As my father used to say when my sisters or I had a setback, this was only a stumble, not a fall. I instructed him to use the weight machines for a week without worrying about how much weight he was lifting, just to get reacquainted with the movements. After that, I would put together another training program for him, and we would set about the task of rebuilding him.

Despite my confidence, Burt was still discouraged. He was sure that we couldn't possibly get back to where we had left off earlier. But I explained to him that as long as the laws of physics, chemistry, and anatomy still apply in our universe, we were sure to climb right back up the fitness ladder. It was just a matter of time. That's the wonder of the human body: give it a reasonable challenge, and it will rise to the occasion.

Burt took my advice, and we resumed our training. Soon, his strength and muscle mass started to return. It was only later that he told me how much my encouragement had helped him through his dark times. Instead of spiraling downward in free fall, he was able to once again take control of his life by having a plan to follow. Fitness wasn't just restoring his body; it was restoring his hope and his faith.

Burt continued to regain his strength, but his battle with his disease also continued. He moved to Boston to be closer to his family. We kept in touch, but then, suddenly, I stopped hearing from him. I found out that Burt had died from his illness. I'm usually very positive and upbeat about life, but I was suddenly filled with a sense of futility. What had it mattered that we had improved his strength 30 percent last year? What was the point of all that hard work?

I began then to think of my high school biochemistry lessons, about the energy bonds that held the electrons of our molecules in their orbits. The solidity of our bodies, of the entire physical world, really, was just an illusion; at the atomic level, there was more empty space than matter. I began to imagine my body—all of our bodies—not as whole organisms, but rather as collections of molecules bound together by only by these energy bonds. What if these molecules suddenly decided to disperse? What if the only thing keeping our atoms from flying apart was our own willpower, our stubborn refusal to cease to exist? How long could any of us be expected to hold these millions of molecules together before we tired and failed?

I began to think of the endless upkeep all of our bodies require to stay in proper trim. Every day, the body needs to be fed, to be trained, to be stretched and washed. The heart beats, the blood flows, and waste is eliminated. Sleep provides some respite, but then the cycle begins again, every day, until we cease to exist.

It was an exhausting thought. I began to imagine an escape from the tyranny of this routine, of a time and place without decay, where there is no struggle to improve and maintain one's collection of molecules. A place where there is no injury, no need to train, no need to run. A place where there is stillness.

I had reached the bottom, a place beyond the marathon, beyond running, beyond wondering about the active life. I had peered into a dark hole where existence itself is questioned. From the Big Bang through the thousands of millennia of

Why Run the Marathon? Second Lap

existence, to the end of time and a return to the stillness from which it all was born, I saw that nothing truly endured but the stillness itself.

I shook off these dark thoughts, recoiling like a child touching a hot oven. Down that hole is a place where existence denies itself. A place without change is a place without the possibility of improvement, without challenge. Because it has neither success nor failure, it is a place without meaning. A place of such stillness is a place of death.

I decided to imagine my body differently. Instead of seeing it on the verge of pulling apart, I see my molecules spinning tightly in their orbits, strengthened and nourished by their numbers and their energy bonds. Every movement strengthens them further, and they shine brighter in the flexing and stretching of my muscles. I returned to solid ground, within the sphere of my experience. This was now familiar to me, because I knew the peaceful fatigue that I felt when I lived the active life; I knew that the joy of exertion conquers the stillness.

My body spoke in one voice, and made its choice. It chose movement, it chose running, it chose the marathon. It chose life. That was enough for now.

To the End of the Earth

When January 1999 rang in, I had been racing for twelve years, and had run a total of 39 marathons. I had run up and down a mountain, and I had qualified for the Boston Marathon. In short, I felt that I was quite experienced. I had become something of a marathon connoisseur; while some people collected art or fine wine, I collected marathons. My collection had a serious flaw, however; I had yet to race away from American soil. That had to change. But I wanted my first race off American soil to be memorable. True to my nature, I wanted it to be *inspiring.* And I found it. After running my 40th marathon in Houston, I picked a jaw-dropping race for my 41st. In fact, I wasn't going to simply run a marathon; I was going to undertake an honest-to-goodness *expedition.* I had signed on for a race at the end of the world. I was going to run the Antarctica Marathon.

To be honest, the idea of running a marathon in Antarctica hadn't been burning in my thoughts. In fact, the idea never even occurred to me until I received a phone call from my friend Ginny Turner, a fellow marathoner who was also pursuing the fifty-state Holy Grail. I had met Ginny in South Bend, Indiana—at a marathon, of course. Standing inside Notre Dame's stadium after crossing the finish line, I explained to her the legendary "Touchdown Jesus," the image of Christ painted larger than life on the side of a building that can be seen from inside the stadium, beyond the goalposts. Some nameless smart-aleck many years ago had noticed how the figure's upraised arms resembled an umpire's signal for a score, and so a legend was born. Ginny and I became fast friends after that, and kept in touch over the following months, comparing marathon notes and schedules. So I wasn't at all surprised when she called me one day to tell me that she was planning to run another marathon. But I never expected to hear that it would be in Antarctica.

Ginny wanted me to join her on the expedition. I was interested, of course, but skeptical. I had been working as an attorney for a decade, but as a government employee, my salary was still low, and I was still saddled with massive student loans to repay. This would be an expensive adventure, and I just didn't think I could manage the cost. But as I opened my mouth to explain to Ginny why I couldn't go, she hit me with her final sales pitch: when she returned later and told me all about the journey, I would realize that I should have gone with her, and would forever regret not going. That stopped me cold. She was absolutely right. I found myself saying yes to her, even as my mind scrambled to figure out a way to pay for it. I got off the phone and signed up for the expedition that was to take place the following month.

Having committed to the race, I thought it would be a good idea to find out exactly what I'd gotten myself into. Once I received the race materials, I settled back for a nice read. The Antarctic Marathon—also called The Last Marathon, because that's the last place a sane person would think of running a race—is held in February, at the height of the austral summer. It was organized by a travel company that catered to marathoners, a reflection of the financial clout of the burgeoning marathon culture. Our group was comprised of over 160 runners from around the world, led by a team of naturalists who would handle technical matters and shore landings, and who would explain this vast wasteland to us.

My journey began with a 10½-hour overnight flight from New York's JFK airport to Buenos Aires. As if that wasn't challenging enough, I managed to arrive at the gate only 15 minutes before departure. This brand of reckless tardiness was, unfortunately, bred in my bones; the rest of my family treats deadlines no more respectfully than I do. Upon my arrival at the gate, the airline staff was both relieved and annoyed to see me, knowing that a member of a large group on the flight was unaccounted for just moments before the doors were to close. In their haste to get me on board, they assigned me to the first available seat they could find. It was in first class. Not really a good incentive for me to correct my errant behavior. Of course, this occurred in the years before the post-9/11 security clampdown, when such last-minute adventures were possible.

After arriving in Buenos Aires and meeting other members of the team, I joined a few of them for a little walk around the city, to shake off the kinks and to get the lay of the land. Getting around Buenos Aires turned out to be easy; it's really a walkers' city, crisscrossed with broad, beautiful boulevards, and filled with beautiful European architecture. Avenida 9 de Julio, at some 600 feet across, is one of the broadest thoroughfares in the world, while Florida and Lavale avenues are open pedestrian malls. We saw tango dancers whirling among street musicians, vendors in the flea market of San Telmo, and one of the copies of Rodin's *Thinker* pondering ceaselessly in front of the Congreso Nacional. Nearby was the beautiful opera house, the Teatro Colón, where Toscanini and Caruso had performed. And, of course, we made our pilgrimage to Eva Perón's tomb in the Recoleta cemetery. The site itself is unremarkable, but the cemetery as a whole is fascinating. It's a virtual city of the dead, filled entirely with mausoleums, each vying to be the most ostentatious.

Being a native New Yorker, however, I also insisted on descending belowground to check out the subway system. I discovered that the stations were like underground cities, containing dozens of small shops and eateries. The platforms were lined with beautiful ceramic murals, and the trains were wood-paneled antiques.

Making our way back to our hotel, we strolled along Puerto Madero, where a canal lined with fine restaurants opens into the Río de la Plata. Couples strolled the promenade, sharing ice cream cones and whispered conversations. When we finally made it back to our hotel room, I fell into my bed and, as my grandmother would have said, slept like the dead.

By the following morning, I was recovered and ready to run. I found the Parque Natural y Zonade Reserva Ecológica Costanera Sur, just east of Puerto Madero, where I did laps on a popular running and cycling circuit: an 8-kilometer hardpack dirt and gravel road that encircled the park. Later, I joined the full team and the travel company staff for a debriefing. In addition to other warnings, the hotel staff cautioned us about a tourist scam that involved one conspirator spraying mustard on an unsuspecting victim, while another conspirator suddenly appears and offers to help clean off the mustard. That's when bandits suddenly appear from nowhere to snatch bags and cameras from the distracted victim, and run off in different directions. This must be a joke, I said, but I was assured that it was true.

As if to prove the point, Ginny and I later got mustarded while wandering around near the Teatro Colon opera house. Although we didn't see who had surreptitiously sprayed us with mustard, we knew what to expect once we saw that we'd suffered a condiment attack, so we ignored offers of "help" from a nearby elderly woman, and quickly walked off before any bandits appeared. I was indignant; I didn't grow up on the streets of Manhattan to get mugged in Buenos Aires!

Finally, it was time to begin the next leg of our journey: a 4½-hour flight south to Patagonia, at the tip of South America. On the way down, strong winds buffeted our plane, and the pilot made an emergency landing to wait out the squalls. We stayed in our seats as the jet shuddered on the tarmac, silently exchanging worried glances among ourselves. Finally, the winds died down, and we returned to the air. As far as I was concerned, this is when the expedition officially began.

Eventually we arrived in a small but beautiful airport, topped with a latticework of timber and glass. We were in Ushuaia, in Argentinean Tierra del Fuego, the land of fire, named for the burning torches along the shore that were spotted by passing sailors. It was an apt name, because it was a dramatic place. The wind blew, the rain fell, clouds drifted in and out, and sometimes the sun even shone—often all within half an hour. The turbulence of the weather was echoed in the forbidding look of the cragged peaks surrounding the city. I had heard the place described as the City at the End of the World, and that seemed appropriate, too. Despite the human footprint on the land, it still appeared primordial.

Ushuaia is small, but it still offered some interesting sights, like the old prison, now open for nonconvict visitors. There was also a large nature preserve, and, most interesting to me, little houses mounted on sleds. As I learned, real estate ownership had been a loose concept at the tip of the world. When a dispute over land occurred, local residents traditionally solved the problem by simply moving their houses across the road. There weren't many of these sled-houses left, though; in Ushuaia, as in so many northern cities, open land was becoming a less and less readily available commodity.

With our time in Ushuaia concluded, our group met on the dock to board one of two chartered Russian research ships for the two-and-a-half day journey south through the treacherous Drake Passage. I had signed on with the smaller ship, which carried forty-six passengers. At this point we met our full expedition staff, led by Shane Evoy, a large, bearded, garrulous man who seemed perfectly suited to his work. The staff seemed to be a fun and enthusiastic bunch. One crew member confided to me that they had been looking forward to seeing us for weeks, since our ultra-fit group was a nice change from the often sedentary, elderly tourists that they usually escort to the Southern Continent.

Along with the expedition staff was the Russian crew who manned the vessel. Not many of them spoke English, but they proved themselves to be very hard-working, prompting me to learn at least one word of Russian: *spaciba*, meaning thank you. We were allowed to go up to the bridge and watch them in action, as long as we kept out of their way. The kitchen staff was equally good, providing three great meals a day, plus snacks. As a bachelor living alone back in the States, I found myself eating better aboard the ship than I did at home.

The ship itself was comfortable, but utilitarian. There was no lido deck or pool, but there was a bar—well-used on our trip—a lecture room, a small library, and even a sauna. Bathrooms and shower stalls were shared, with plenty of hot water available. The cabins were wood-paneled, each with two closets and a desk. Bunks had reading lights and curtains for privacy. Laundry service was available on the ship as well, though that seemed to be the kind of extra frill this group wouldn't go for. We thought ourselves hardier stock than that.

As part of the prerace package, I received an informational guidebook, which I devoured along with a score of other books on the history and environment of the White Continent. Once on the ship, I watched films and attended lectures offered by the expedition's naturalists. Surprisingly it wasn't hard to get a feel for the place. Antarctica, I learned, had no indigenous people, and was populated only by whales, penguins, seals, a few species of birds, and the shrimplike krill on which many of the other animals fed. Not much of anything, really.

Still, Antarctica proved fascinating in the way a simple, pure color on canvas can be captivating. But I couldn't help viewing all of the information I came across through the eyes of a runner, so when I read about air avalanches, called *katabatic winds*, I felt myself gritting my teeth. While most wind is caused by differences in air pressure, these winds are caused instead by gravity. Just as hot air rises, cold air can fall, and in Antarctica, cold air sometimes falls so rapidly that it can blow at 40 mph or more. I knew that if this occurred during my race, there wouldn't be much I could do about it other than lean in and fight like hell. As I read about those winds, I suddenly realized that nothing I had done before—including Pikes Peak—had really prepared me for what I might find down here on race day.

No Antarctic education is complete, of course, without learning the story of exploration. The tales of courage, suffering and vanity left me awestruck. Especially memorable was the Shackleton expedition. Ernest Shackleton set out in 1914 on the aptly named *Endurance* to become the first man to traverse the Antarctic continent, the South Pole having already been won. Before he even managed to reach land, however, his ship became ice-locked. All efforts to free the ship failed, and by late 1915, the shifting mass of ice had crushed his ship, leaving the crew to live on the ice with three lifeboats and whatever supplies they were able to salvage from the *Endurance* before it went under. Eventually, the ice broke up, and the crew took to the lifeboats and made their way through rough seas and freezing weather to a spit of rock called Elephant Island.

Their new home was well outside any established shipping lanes, and realizing that their chances for rescue were slim—and recognizing, too, that a steady diet of nothing but penguin meat was taking a terrible toll on his crew—Shackleton set out with a few handpicked men in one of the lifeboats to find help. In what has been hailed as one of the all-time greatest feats of seamanship, Shackleton managed to steer his 22-foot open boat 800 nautical miles through wild and freezing seas to King George Island, where there was a whaling station. But the currents had forced Shackleton to land on the far side of the island, and now he and his crew had to scale uncharted mountains to reach the station. Once again, Shackleton accomplished the impossible, and after they stumbled into town, the station's captain could scarcely believe the tale that the ragged, unshaven, exhausted band of men told him. By August 1916, Shackleton managed to secure a ship and rescue his crew. All hands made it back home alive.

Lying back in my warm and comfortable bunk, I could scarcely believe such a thing had ever happened. But there was a postscript to the story. When Shackleton returned to England, he expected to be hailed as a hero, but in his absence all of Europe had been embroiled in the bloodbath known as the Great War. Faced with the story of men who risked their lives for adventure and glory, and who lived to tell the tale, a weary and grief-stricken public gave a collective shrug. Shackleton's agonies paled in comparison to the tragedies *they* had endured.

Somehow, I felt an odd kinship with Shackleton. He set out to face suffering—perhaps not as much as he bargained for, but guaranteed suffering nonetheless—when it would have been just as easy and acceptable to stay home. Although his aim was clearly fame and fortune, I felt that there must have been something more to make the deprivation worthwhile: a desire, a need, to test his own limits. That much resonated with me. I knew that I, too, valued suffering for its own sake, though mostly just in 26.2-mile doses.

Our ship made its way from Ushuaia through the Beagle Channel into open water, escorted by Magellanic penguins swimming below, and albatross soaring above. After rounding Cape Horn, we entered the dreaded Drake Passage, where the Atlantic and the Pacific oceans converge to create the roughest seas on Earth. Waves routinely crest there at 25 to 30 feet, and often higher. For me, surviving the Drake was the biggest challenge of the trip. I never had what you would call a strong stomach, and I was well aware of the irony of my being on a ship on high seas after a lifetime of enduring queasiness on ferries and carnival rides.

I hadn't come unarmed. I'd prepared for the "Drake Shake" with every antinausea treatment known to science, and a few others besides. My doctor provided me with antinausea scopolamine patches, my pharmacist provided me with acupressure wristbands and old-fashioned Dramamine, and an herbalist sold me ginger candies to settle my stomach. I also knew that gazing at a stable point on the distant horizon while breathing deep gulps of fresh air would be helpful. With all these remedies in my bag of tricks, I felt as ready as I could possibly be.

I was surprised, then, and even a bit disappointed, to find that the seas were calm. Instead of the Drake Shake, we got the Drake Lake. All that worrying for nothing. With such calm waters, I was even able to get in a workout, ducking though portholes and sliding around the corners of the deck as I ran for 45 minutes. Several team members joined in, and we quickly dubbed our workout the Drake 5K. Much to our delight, we were told by the expedition staff that the Russian crew thought we were crazy.

After two-and-a-half days of listening to lectures, socializing at the bar, and gazing out at the horizon, we finally saw a few bits of sea ice. Then we had our first glimpse of land. We were out of the Drake Passage and were approaching the South Shetland Islands, just off the Antarctic Peninsula. It was summer in Antarctica, but the temperature was still in the 20s and low 30s, with gusting winds bringing it down into the teens. We all dug out our waterproof gear as the expedition staff prepared for our first landing. There weren't any docks or piers to welcome us, so all landings were wet. After scampering down a gangway, we climbed ten at a time into inflated, motorized boats called Zodiacs, which were driven as far up onto the rocky beach as possible. One by one, we swung our legs over the side and charged the surf like soldiers at Normandy. After experiencing this landing, I understood why we had each been required to acknowledge in writing that we were not guaranteed a marathon; if bad weather made a wet landing hazardous, there would be no race.[2]

When I first signed up for the expedition, the tour company director told me that although I was coming down to Antarctica for the marathon, it would slip into lesser significance when compared to everything else I would see down there. He was right. Our first stop was a visit to the Polish scientific base camp, followed by a landing at a penguin rookery, where thousands of Chinstrap and Gentoo penguins mingled about, molting and nesting. Following the staff's directions, we sat very still, and soon the cute, impossibly clumsy little guys came right up to us, climbing onto our laps and nibbling on our pant legs. I captured their cooing and braying on a micro tape recorder, which I thought would provide a perfect soundtrack for slide shows back home. All of this was wonderful, but one thing was not: the smell. These were wild animals, after all, and when they crowd together in one place by the thousands, there were bound to be repercussions.

Not so different from runners at a starting line, actually.

After making several other Zodiac landings, including one to the ruins of a former whaling station at Deception Island, we finally made our way to King George Island, where the staff laid out our marathon course. It was to be a double figure-8 loop, and it was every bit as difficult as we imagined it would be. The first loop of the figure 8 (which would also be the third loop as I made my way around the course for the second time), was a 1½-mile run across a rocky beach, up the side of a glacier, and back. We would then run along rough dirt roads and across a frigid stream past several scientific bases.

---

2 In fact, in the very next Antarctic Marathon expedition, held two years later, a landing was not possible. Nonetheless, in a feat that could be described as either monumentally determined or frighteningly compulsive, a marathon was held onboard the ship, consisting of 420 laps around the deck. Let's just say that I'm glad that I didn't have to consider that option.

This island, and indeed, this entire frozen continent, is governed by the Antarctic Treaty system, which provides that while no country may claim sovereignty over these lands or engage in commercial exploitation of its natural resources, countries may establish scientific bases to conduct research. A human presence is especially evident on King George Island, where seven nations built small villages. Our group was hosted by the Uruguayans, and their base would mark the start and finish of the race.

On race day, we awoke early and ate breakfast. The waters were calm, so we were able to land without incident. We were allowed into the small dining hall in the Uruguayan base to prepare ourselves for the race, but because their living space was modest, we weren't allowed to keep any of our bags inside the building. It was a small inconvenience, and no one seemed to mind. We also had to provide our own water bottles, which the staff placed out on the course for us.

As we lined up for the start of the race, I saw that several of the local residents had taken up the tour leader's offer to join us for the race. Most striking was an older, plump Russian woman who wore running shorts, a T-shirt, and oven mitts instead of the tights, long sleeve shirts, jackets and running gloves that the rest of us wore. Clearly, improvisation is a crucial skill down there.

The starting signal was given—a horn blare from a megaphone—and we dashed across the broken rock toward the glacier. I had expected that its surface would be a slippery sheet of ice, but instead I found it to more like an ice chip mountain. That made it not only more treacherous than I was expecting, but also prone to suddenly giving way, leaving a runner knee-deep in a previously hidden hole. Cracks in the ice only compounded the problem, making for very slow going.

After reaching the turnaround point on top of the glacier, and smiling for the official race cameraman, I carefully made my way back down past the Uruguayan base, and then continued along rough dirt roads, over steep hills, and past a small lake, toward the Chilean base and on to the Chinese and the Russian bases that lay beyond. I later learned that one member of our team stopped into the Chinese base, where he bartered for a watch and was treated to a warm drink.

Not being as creative, I just focused on the race. A spot of warm weather created mud fields for us to slog through, as curious penguins watched closely. There was something eerily magnetic about the penguins; I saw more than one runner veer off course toward them, as if hypnotized. A few shouts brought them back to their senses and to the racecourse. More perilous, though, were the skuas: big, darkly colored birds that were reported to be fiercely protective of their nests. If we wandered too close to one of their nests, we were told, a skua would swoop down and attack us. The problem, though, was that their nests weren't always in plain view. At one point on the course several of us apparently came too close, because a skua took wing and made repeated dives at us, which we warded off by wildly swinging our arms.

After more than five hours of sliding, mucking, hiking, and even running across the Antarctic tundra, I finally crossed the finish line. Marathon number 41 was in the books. I was neither the first nor the last runner to finish. Since the fancy new trail shoes I had brought had given me some nasty blisters, I was perfectly happy to have just made it through the whole way. We returned to our ship to clean up, nap, and fill our bellies, and then were transported to the larger ship for an onboard awards presentation.

The following day, we set off for another highlight: our dramatic landing on the Antarctic mainland itself. We boarded the Zodiac boats again, and made out way to a landing on the Antarctic Peninsula. It was similar to the other landings we had made, but somehow, it felt different. Gazing at the rock and ice around us, I think we all felt that we were finally, truly, at the bottom of the world, at one of the last unspoiled expanses left on Earth. I wondered whether our brand of ecotourism was helping to build political support to preserve it, or whether, despite our precautions and good intentions, we were the beginning of a flood of tourists who would unwittingly destroy it.[3] Our usually rambunctious group had fallen into silence; I supposed that they were all wondering the same thing.

And then it was back through the Drake. This time the seas were not so friendly, as the ship pitched and rolled through 35- and 40-foot waves. We were banned from the outside deck, as well as the bridge. Digging deep into my bag of tricks, I managed to keep my insides inside and my stomach quiet, provided that I stayed prone in my bed. Strangely enough, the same corkscrewing, rolling action that slammed me from wall to wall and turned my stomach when I tried walking felt comforting once I lay down. I decided not to fight it; I buried myself under my covers, and drifted off to sleep, rocked by the southern ocean like a baby in a crib.

Two days later we landed in Ushuaia, and few days after that I was standing in a terminal at JFK airport in New York City. It was snowing, and the temperature was near zero—colder, in fact, than it was just then in Antarctica. I stood for a few minutes off to the side of the arrival gate, trying to adjust to the sudden noise and bustle. I had never before felt so different from everyone else.

---

3 My fears were, unfortunately, well-founded. In November 2007, the cruise ship *MS Explorer* sank in Antarctica. While all 154 passengers and crew were rescued, the ship left behind a mile-long oil spill that could not be immediately cleaned up because of bad weather. As scientists worried about the effect of the spill on the 2,500 penguins who were about to pass that area, the Argentinean government announced that it was considering limiting the level of ecotourism to the area.

Running Tip #6

Preparing for Antarctica

- *Don't bother with speed work.* The Antarctic Marathon isn't for PRs, so instead, concentrate training on hills and trails.
- *Bring the right clothing.* Dress in layers: running tights, a long sleeve wicking top, and lightweight running gloves to keep warm, covered by wind pants, a lightweight water-resistant running jacket, and lightweight water-resistant gauntlet mittens over your gloves. Shed clothing cautiously, since the wind could suddenly pick up and the temperature drop.
- *Bring the right gear.* Use trail shoes, gaiters (short, protective ankle sleeves that help keep out dirt and water), and mini-crampons (rubber outsoles with short, plastic spikes for better traction on ice).
- *Bring a disposable, panoramic camera.* After all, this is a once-in-a-lifetime kind of race.

Finally: Boston!

After returning home from Antarctica, I felt oddly depressed. For the first time as a runner, I felt unmotivated. I realized that Antarctica was to blame. I had harbored so much anticipation for the race that once it was over, I felt let down. The Boston Marathon was coming up in just two months, and I couldn't afford a training slump. To properly prepare for Boston, I needed another marathon to restore my motivation and keep me in prime condition. That's how I came to run the 1999 Los Angeles Marathon.

Signing up for the race was the easy part, but I was a bit sloppy on figuring out the logistics. I had traveled alone to run the race, and ended up staying in a hotel about 8 miles or so from the race start. I took a taxi to the race packet pick-up the day before the marathon, which was located near the race start, and was surprised to see how expensive the cab ride would be. Not wanting to blow my budget on transportation, I researched bus routes, and discovered that one bus would drop me off right next to the start. Perfect. The following morning I got up early and waited at the stop next to my hotel. I had given myself plenty of time—unusual for me, but I didn't want to take any chances. Finally, the bus came, and I settled back for a relaxing ride. Everything was under control.

And then, suddenly, there was chaos. The bus pulled over and the driver announced that this was as far as the bus would go, due to street closings caused by the marathon. How could I not have realized this would happen? Anger and frustration boiled up inside me, stoked by the realization that we were still about six miles from the race start, with precious little time to spare before the gun.

No need to panic, yet; I just had to hail a cab, and everything would be okay. I began walking down the street in search of a taxi. I quickly realized, though, that the streets were deserted due to the street closings. All I saw were traffic cones and occasional police cruisers. Checking my watch, I saw that there were just 5 minutes until the race start. It was time to panic. I broke into a run, scouring each street that I passed for signs of life. I picked up the pace, and went into top gear. I knew this wasn't the way to warm up for a marathon, but I had little choice.

Finally, I saw a cab, and was able to flag it down. I explained my situation to him, and he zipped off to the freeway, promising to get me to the race. We had just a few scant minutes, and six miles to go. I anxiously counted the passing seconds as we weaved through traffic. With my eyes glued to my watch, I saw the official starting time come and go. We were still on the highway. I was heartbroken. My driver reassured me that we were close, and as we neared the start downtown, I told him to just pull over. I threw money toward the front seat and leapt out of the cab, scrambled up the embankment, and hurtled over the guardrail. In front of me was the starting area, now bereft of all runners. The race was already 10 minutes old. People were milling about, and workers had started taking down the starting sign. This race was not turning out to be a good motivator for running Boston the following month!

"Runner coming through!" I yelled, dodging and weaving through the crowd. Up ahead, an electronic mat straddled the street, activated by a chip containing a transponder that each runner fixed to his or her shoe. Most big races use these to track runners and record each runner's finishing time. As I crossed the starting line, the very last person to do so in a field of more than 10,000 runners, I heard a reassuring beep. I was officially in the race.

Starting dead last has its benefits, as I soon learned. Usually the ranks of runners in a big race are shoulder to shoulder for the first mile or so, until they begin to spread out. It's only then that you can settle into your own target race pace. Not so for the last-place runner, however. From my vantage point, I could see that the field had already spread, and I was able to run as fast as I wanted from the very start. I began to wonder if this might not be a good way to intentionally start my races, but I quickly put that thought out of my head. Like a dog ordered to sit still while a juicy steak was inches from its nose, I knew that I wouldn't be able to fight off the urge to run once the gun goes off in a race and everyone surges forward. I was disciplined enough to run the marathon, but not disciplined enough to not run it, even for ten minutes.

I soon discovered another great benefit to starting in the back; you get to pass people. You get to pass *a lot* of them, and that's a good feeling. But more than that, you get to really see the race; I saw people who would usually be invisible to me, buried in sea of humanity far behind me. Among these faces in Los Angeles were several runners I knew from other races, people I didn't even know were planning to run L.A. If I hadn't started in the back of the pack, I never would have seen them, and never would have had a chance to say hello. It was a rare and welcome treat.

When all was said and done, I crossed the finish line in L.A. with a good time, and a story to boot. Marathon number 42 was history. And better still, I had restored my desire to race. I was like a lion pacing in a cage, and Boston was the meat laid in front of me.

Boston had always seemed like a dream to me, like a Camelot for runners, more myth than reality. I had run it once before as a charity fund-raiser, but that didn't feel right to me. Not to take anything away from all those dedicated and caring runners who race as fund-raisers—many of whom I coached myself—getting my Boston race number without running a qualifying time was hollow for me because I hadn't *earned it*. But in April 1999, I had earned my spot officially. From the barren waste-land of Antarctica to the famous starting line of the Boston Marathon in the outlying town of Hopkinton, I was on quite a roll.

From the moment I arrived in town, I couldn't help but get swept up in the excitement. While other cities sometimes ignore or tolerate their marathons, Boston is absolutely in love with theirs, and it showed. Banners and signs advertising the race were everywhere. Stores offered marathon merchandise—and not just the running stores—and seemingly everyone I met asked if I was running the race. Strangers smiled and wished me luck. Suddenly, marathoning wasn't a fringe sport, it was front-page news.

The runners themselves flooded the streets, shops, and restaurants like locusts. There was an audible buzz in the air, made up of dozens of simultaneous conversations about training, about the racecourse, and about qualifying races. The Boston Marathon began to feel like it was something more than a race; it began to feel like a mass movement.

And that, of course, is what it is. Any doubts were dispelled at packet pickup at the cavernous convention center, where thousands of people lined up to get their race numbers and to check out the expo. At most races, packet pickup is often little more than a quick, prerace chore, but here it's an *event*, a celebration of life and of running. Just making it into Boston is an achievement, and being part of the race said something about a person's work ethic and lifestyle.

Even the official Boston Marathon shirt made a statement. It was devoid of any splashy multi-color race emblem, and it lacked the tangle of corporate sponsor logos that covered most other race shirts. In Boston, you always get a long-sleeved shirt with a small Boston Athletic Association logo on the breast and *Boston Marathon* written down one arm. The color of the shirt varies from year to year, but the design never changes. It's quiet and dignified, and there's no other running shirt like it.

After picking up my race packet, I wandered around the expo. The energy was unbelievable. There was a palpable excitement in the air, heightened by the presence of so many of the world's greatest runners, past and present, signing autographs and talking with fans. In contrast to many professional athletes in other sports, these pros were friendly and accessible, swapping stories, training tips, and race strategies with anyone they met. I wondered whether this easy rapport stemmed from the fact that on race day, we would all face the same challenge. While even the most rabid Red Sox fan would likely never dig in at the plate at Fenway Park, any runner of any ability can go head-to-head against the best runners in the world by simply entering a race. Even Boston, with its qualifying times, provides a place where runners of modest ability can mix with the elite. And on race day, we have a shared experience: we all have to handle the weather, the course, and the challenge of covering the miles as fast as we can. It's a leveling experience.

Perhaps, too, the difference between running and other sports lies in the basis for excellence. While all top athletes train and practice, runners rely mostly on the relentless grind of their training, and not on any superior hand-eye coordination, as baseball and basketball players do. Elite runners are genetically gifted, sure, but without intense training, those gifts are wasted. Their training creates a strong work ethic that leaves humility in its wake. There are no short cuts in marathoning, so anyone who is a marathoner has worked hard. It's a lesson no one forgets.

After a few hours, I had had enough of the expo, and staggered out with a bag of promos, giveaways, premiums, and samples. I ate an early prerace meal, and spent the next few hours lying sleeplessly in bed. Finally, it was race day. Not Sunday morning, though, as it would be with most races, but Monday, the state holiday known as Patriot's Day. In Boston, that means a day off, a Red Sox game, and the Marathon.

Getting to the marathon was an adventure in itself. The Boston Marathon, like marathons in New York City, Las Vegas, and numerous other places, uses a point-to-point course. This turns the marathon into a true journey, as runners pass from town to town, along country roads, over train tracks, into the heart of the city. The problem, though, is that unlike loop or out-and-back courses, runners don't return to where they started. This creates a logistical challenge: thousands of runners have to be transported from downtown Boston out to the start line, where water, shelter, and bathrooms are provided for them as they wait several hours for the last of the participants to arrive. I'm sure race morning is a mad scramble for the race staff, but for the runners, it's an exercise in rushing to do nothing, and it can be quite frustrating.

Most point-to-point races require a predawn lineup for bus transport. In Boston, the race doesn't begin until noon, and the wait at the high school in Hopkinton—transformed into the Athletes' Village on race day—can be three hours or more.[4] This is my least favorite part of the marathon experience. I've learned to deal with it, and I've even found some ways to make the process a bit more tolerable. At the New York City Marathon one year, instead of waiting on line with other runners for the bus to starting area in Staten Island, some friends of mine and I rented a limo to drop us off at the starting line. It felt decadent, but split between us, it really wasn't too expensive at all, and not only did we avoid the predawn bus lines and were able to sleep a little bit later, but we were able to enjoy the envious and curious stares from other runners as we emerged from our ride.

In Boston, though, I wasn't so lucky or creative. I waited on one of the many long lines at Boston Commons as the fleet of yellow school

---

4 In 2007, years of tradition were abandoned as the race was moved up to 10 A.M. to avoid the worst of the midday heat that had plagued runners in the preceding few years.

buses made their circuit to the race start and back. Eventually, I boarded one of the buses, and settled into a window seat. As the bus droned and rocked, I fell into a drowsy stupor. Finally we arrived at our base camp. Rows of Porta-Jons and several big tents had been set up on the school grounds, along with a stage where various speakers and musicians provided information, advice, and entertainment. My drowsiness quickly disappeared, both from a sudden adrenaline rush and from the shock of cold air. April is a tricky time in Massachusetts; it could be scorching hot or icy cold, but no matter which it is, the chances are that at some point you'll be uncomfortable on race day. That year, it was cold, which made waiting for the race to begin an awful ordeal.

Well, not entirely awful. There was one special marathon tradition that I witnessed and would never forget: the moment marathon legend Johnny Kelley took the stage. Kelley first ran the Boston Marathon in 1928, and won the race in 1935 and 1945. He finished in second place seven times, and was in the top ten eighteen times. He also competed in the 1936 Olympic Games, but he was perhaps more famous for holding the record for the number of times he'd entered the Boston Marathon (sixty-one), and the number of times he finished it (fifty-eight). He was also immortalized in the 1936 race, when eventual winner Tarzan Brown (and how's that for a name!) passed him on the last of three brutal hills in the town of Newton, a moment, the press reported, that broke Kelley's heart. That hill would forevermore be known as Heartbreak Hill, and would eventually be the site of a statue depicting a young Johnny Kelley running hand in hand with an older version of himself.

As I stood before the stage in Hopkinton that morning, Kelley looked thin and frail, a vestige of the great athlete that he once was. Then he spoke. He told us to enjoy the day, to be careful on the course, and to enjoy ourselves. Finding a reserve of strength, as he must have done all those times on Heartbreak Hill, Kelley asked if we'd like him to sing for us. We all clapped and cheered, and Kelley broke into his signature song,

"Young At Heart." The crowd went crazy, laughing and applauding, as cameras clicked all around me. Everyone seemed to recognize that this was one of those special moments, one we would carry with us and share with others for many years to come.[5]

After several hours, we were called away from the school and out onto the street, where corrals had been roped off to separate runners according to their expected finishing times. Standing around for hours drinking water, coffee, and sports drink—as nasty a combination as I could think of—had taken its toll on many of the runners, but the good folks of Hopkinton didn't seem very sympathetic to our plight. Many homeowners patrolled their bushes like guard dogs, shouting away any runners who tried to take care of business surreptitiously. Rather unfriendly, I thought, but what did I know? I lived in a condo, and knew zilch about gardening. For all I knew, the cumulative effects of 18,000 or so overly hydrated, nervous runners could lead to permanent deforestation, so I tried to be sensitive to the concerns of the local community.

The excitement grew as noon approached. Then finally, after years of dreaming, months of planning, hours of waiting, we were off. The Boston Marathon had begun!

The cheering at the starting line was incredible, as the runners passed through a gauntlet of spectators and tried to settle down into their pace. The Boston Marathon is really a tour through a series of towns, which the marathon fanatics can recite in order: *Hopkinton—Ashland—Natick—Wellesley—Newton—Brookline—Boston.* Strategically, this presents some interesting possibilities. Most people focus on the big hills of Newton, stacked one after another between miles 17 and 21, where runners have just started feeling deep fatigue and doubt. What most people don't really consider, however, is that the Boston Marathon is actually a

---

5 Johnny Kelley last ran the Boston Marathon in 1992, when he was eighty-four. He died on October 6, 2004, at the age of ninety-seven.

very fast course, dropping 413 feet over the first 17 miles. Over the next 4 miles, in Newton, runners must climb back up 187 feet, but then the course drops another 127 feet from Newton to the finish line. Apart from those difficult hills in Newton, then, the Boston Marathon is mostly a downhill course.

So, what to do? Conventional wisdom is to run the first 17 downhill miles conservatively and save energy for Newton. Once those big hills are conquered, it would be time to turn on the gas and fly through the final 5 miles to the finish. That was the way Boston was supposed to be run.

Naturally, I decided to do something different. My problem with the conventional wisdom was that the miles before Newton represented two-thirds of the whole race. If I ran that part conservatively, then even if I felt great in the last 5 miles and ran that section hard, I wouldn't be able to make up for all those mediocre early miles, and I would wind up with a mediocre finishing time. On the other hand, if I ran those first 17 miles hard, and struggled through the hills of Newton, I would have only 5 miles between myself and the finish line. I would no doubt be dog tired at that point, but if I could just muster up a little more courage and manage to hold onto my pace, I could wind up with a great finishing time.

Or, I could blow up, and find my body in full revolt in Newton, leaving me sprawled on the grass on the side of the road, exhausted and broken.

Those were basically my options as I saw them. Dare greatly and risk dropping out, or run conservative toward a good, if not glorious, finish.

I thought back to the words of the late Steve Prefontaine, probably the greatest middle-distance runner the United States has ever produced. Pre would often flout conventional wisdom by running out front instead of biding his time for a strong finish. In the 1972 Olympic Games, he pushed the pace in the 5K, running a courageous race but ultimately finishing fourth. "A lot of people run a race to see who's the fastest," he said. "I run to see who has the most guts." That's how I wanted to run. I couldn't win in Boston, of course, but I would run as courageously as anyone there.

With that settled, I streaked through Hopkinton, weaving my way through the runners and enjoying the loud encouragement of the fans packing the roadsides. My legs felt fresh and strong, with lots of pop. In the words of the old Irish toast—appropriate in Boston—it felt as though the road were rising up to greet me. I recognized Darryl, a fellow runner from my track group in D.C. I shouted hello as I flew past. I was running well, and enjoying myself.

The sights of the marathon came and went. I flew past the clock tower in Ashland, the old train station in Framingham, and approached Wellesley. I had heard other runners joking about the enthusiastic co-eds there, but I wasn't prepared for the sheer bedlam of it all. Row upon row of women screamed out to us, offering us encouragement along with offers of kisses. Some guys grinningly took them up on their offers and received a peck, but I was too shy even for that. And, of course, I still had my race to run.

Next up was fabled Newton, and I knew this was where my race would truly begin. If I could make it through the three hills of Newton without breaking, I would have a chance at a great finish.

I hit the first hill, and rode it as the course turned onto broad Commonwealth Avenue. The climb was over a mile long, but I kept my legs churning, and finally I crested the top. The next mile was a gentle downhill, giving all of us a chance to recover our strength and determination for the next challenge ahead. The runners around me were silent, their faces held tight. They seemed like fishermen sailing into a squall, determined not to break. We rode the next hill the same way.

And then Heartbreak Hill was upon us like a storm. Runners swung their arms and fought to hold their pace, grunting and breathing heavily. The crowds were thick along the street and in the broad, grassy median, screaming and waving banners and signs. They knew that this was the most dramatic part of the race, because it was here that the race was usually won and lost; the finish was only for the coronation. And it was here, too, that the humanity and courage of the runners was most evident. We spoke to each another, offering encouragement, trying to share our energy, hoping that together we could bring everyone to the top. A stranger looked over at me and said, "Run with me. We can do this. Run with me."

I pushed to keep up with him, repeating the mantra, "We're almost there, we're almost there, we're almost there." I saw the hilltop just up ahead, and I lowered my eyes. It was so far away, and the road was so steep. I counted off ten seconds before I looked up again. The top of the hill still seemed so distant. I looked back down. Finally, I was there, at the top. I had conquered Heartbreak Hill. I had slowed, but not by very much, and now I just had to pick up the pace and race to the finish in Copley Square.

But did I have anything left in my legs?

I took a moment's breather, and then tried to accelerate. There was that moment's gap, that briefest moment between the command my mind gave, and the response of my legs. I lived a lifetime in that moment, fearful that my legs would refuse to answer my call. But they did. They had not abandoned me. I streaked down the back side of the hill, with renewed strength and hope.

Soon, the excitement of Newton faded behind me, and with it, the adrenaline rush that conquering the hills had given me. There were still 5 miles left to go, and that was a very long way to run on tired legs. I tried to focus only on the patch of road in front of me, and concentrated on maintaining my pace.

I streaked down Commonwealth Avenue, along the train line, and looked up for the massive neon Citgo gas sign in Kenmore Square that would tell me that the finish line was only a mile away. Seeing the sign would be like spotting a lighthouse in a storm at sea; it was the promise of safety, of release from pain and fatigue.

Suddenly, someone jumped in from the crowd and began to match me, stride for stride. It was Lynn, a teammate from my Antarctica adventure. We had kept in touch, and since she lived nearby, she said she'd come to Boston and try to run me in to the finish line. Now there she was, when I needed her most. She didn't have to say much as she ran with me, but I drew energy from her, taking strength from her companionship. I ran like a machine now, thinking only about keeping my legs moving, pushing, pushing, pushing, concentrating on nothing but running.

Finally, the course veered away from Commonwealth Avenue and turned right onto Hereford Street for a couple of blocks, and then left onto Boylston Street. The finish line was just up ahead now. I could see it. It was just a few blocks away. I only had a minute of running left, I told myself. After all these hours, just one single minute. I told myself that I could endure any kind of pain for just one minute. I pushed as hard as I could, sprinting toward the finish line. Lynn matched me, and then drifted away as I flew through the finish line.

I had run the Boston Marathon in 3 hours, 9 minutes, just a single heartbeat slower than my personal best. In the process, I also requalified to run the Boston Marathon the following year. Most importantly, though, I had run courageously, and I felt like I truly belonged at Boston. In this, my 43rd marathon, near the halfway point to reaching my 100-marathon quest, I finally felt like a marathoner.

There was another thing about Boston that was auspicious. I hadn't kept in touch with too many of my old high school friends, but I'd heard through the grapevine, such as it was, that one of our classmates, Stephanie Kay, was teaching art at Boston University. Stephanie and I had been friends in school. We were not very close friends, but I always thought that we got along well. I liked her, but I thought that she was perhaps a little out of my league. She was very pretty, and being an artist, she hung out with the cool crowd. But we were adults now, and I was curious about what she looked like and how she was doing. I left her a message through her office, just letting her know that I was coming into town for the race and would love to catch up with her. I didn't hear back. Well, that was all right. It had been well over a decade since we'd last seen each other, and my message had come out of the blue, so I couldn't blame her for tossing it aside. I guessed that she just wasn't interested.

It would be a while until I found out how wrong I was.

Running Tip #7

Massage

Nonrunners assume that it's better to run downhill than up, but that's not always true. Downhill is *faster*, but it's far more brutal than uphill. After crossing the finish line in Boston, my joints stiffened and my muscles began to ache from all the pounding my body had absorbed. The quadriceps muscles on the front of my legs, which had kept me from falling right on my face, were totally shot. A few days' rest didn't bring much relief. I needed help. I was ready for a massage.

Hard training and racing causes micro-tears and the accumulation of waste products in muscle cells. Adhesions also can occur, in which muscles cells stick together, limiting flexibility and healing. Massage forces waste out of the muscle tissue and breaks up adhesions, resulting in reduced recovery time, improved range of motion, and a lower occurrence of injury.

It can take a while for the benefits of massage to become fully apparent, although the results could sometimes be very dramatic. Once, a massage therapist was working deeply (and painfully!) on a spot in my upper back where I'd been feeling pain, when I suddenly broke out in a drenching sweat. The therapist said it was common for stressed bodies to release their tension that way, and it really did feel as though a clenched fist had suddenly opened up. I felt better immediately.

But don't get massage only when you're injured; aim to get a massage monthly, or even biweekly or weekly if you can afford it. Or try self-massage: knead and rub your target muscles deeply, stroking toward your heart, using massage oil to reduce friction. There are also products available to facilitate self-massage, such as a rolling-pin like device that works especially well on hamstrings and quads.

Across the Pond and Around the World

After conquering Antarctica, traveling abroad for a marathon didn't seem to be such a far-fetched idea. Following Boston, I ran the Salt Lake City Marathon in Utah. Even though I had raced to the top of Pikes Peak, I had never run an entire race at altitude before, and it seemed to have an effect on me that I hadn't anticipated: I suddenly developed an endless need to pull over to the bushes. I had never experienced anything like it before, and I don't know why it happened, but the result was that I was alternately passing and getting passed by the same handful of runners. Finally, one of them had had enough, and as I emerged from the woods for what must have been the tenth time, he yelled out "stop passing me!" All I could do was sheepishly apologize.

Next was an uneventful marathon in Tupelo, Mississippi—uneventful for me, though not for Dave, who joined me for that race. While I flew down for the race, Dave opted to minimize costs by taking an overnight bus down. At one rest stop, he lost track of time, and watched in alarm as his bus pulled out without him on board, but with all his racing gear sitting neatly on his window seat. He hopped the next bus and gave chase. Luckily, this new bus was an express, and he overtook his gear at the next major stop. After all that, running the race was easy for him. Once the race was over, Dave and I decided to go have lunch and celebrate with a few beers. The lunch was easy to find, but not the beer; we couldn't find any place to serve us alcohol on a Sunday. Tough lesson for a city boy like me to learn!

Following Mississippi, I set my sights on Berlin for marathon number 46. Berlin was a city in transition, ground zero for the collapse of communism and the birth of a new Europe. I read about how the city was rebuilding itself and was bristling with energy and excitement. The racecourse was supposed to be a very flat and fast course—several marathon world records had been set there. It seemed like the perfect marathon adventure.

I managed to talk two of my running friends into going with me. Our flights went smoothly, and we checked into our hotel without a problem. We also made it to the packet pickup easily enough; the Berlin Marathon is a huge race, with 20,000 or so participants, so all we had to do was get close to the race headquarters and look for people in running shoes toting their race packets and the goodie bags. We made our way to the great hall and collected our paperwork, only to discover that the race instructions were written only in German.

It's my conceit as an American that no matter where I go, I expect the locals to speak English, and that all instructions will be translated for my convenience. Apparently, the Germans had different ideas on the subject. I scanned the runner instructions. Some of the words bore a passing resemblance to English, but others were just a maze of letters. I was baffled by the German propensity to take lots of small words and mash them together into mammoth tongue twisters. Luckily, the materials had a similar layout to American race instructions, so we were able to more or less figure things out.

However odd and unsettling packet pickup had felt, race morning seemed as familiar and comfortable as an old shirt. Runners gathered at the starting line and did what runners everywhere do; they ate energy bars, drank water, stretched, napped, talked, paced, worried, and relaxed. Eventually, they huddled close together behind the starting line, and then exploded forward en masse at the blast of the starting gun. I found myself part of a teeming, sweating mass pouring through the Brandenburg Gate. It was unforgettable. I was surprised, though, to see mile markers popping up more often than I expected. I checked my last split time—the pace in which I'd run my last mile. My watch read 3:44. That would put me right about at the world record for the mile. *That can't be right*, I thought. Then it dawned on me. *Kilometers.* Those markers measure *kilometers*, not miles. The world record was safe, and worse yet, I would have to pass another 41 of those markers before I was through.

I immediately understood the downside of measuring a marathon course in kilometers—when I see a sign that reads "26," my body knows, like one of Pavlov's dogs, that it has only another minute and a half or so of running, and then it's quitting time. Not so in a European marathon. Marker 26 only tells me that I have another 16 kilometers to go. It's a definite downer.

On the other hand, kilometer markers fly past quicker than mile markers, which gives the feeling of progress being made. It's also an ego boost to pass numbers that get so staggeringly high: 35, 36, 37! On a practical level, having such a profusion of markers also provides runners with more opportunities to check their pace and make any necessary adjustments.

I also discovered anew that a marathon is a splendid way to tour a city. Anyone can lay out a 5K or 10K race course to avoid the seamier sides of a city, but a marathon exposes all there really is to see, the warts along with the beauty. In Berlin, we snaked our way over to the former East Germany, and what I saw there startled me. I had grown up during the Cold War, and had imagined East Germany as the formidable industrial muscle of the Soviet bloc, churning out weapons and superior athletes.

What I saw was no mighty enemy; the buildings all seemed shoddy and in disrepair. If ever this had been a place bustling with energy, that time had long since passed. I felt like I had peeked behind the curtain looking for the Wizard of Oz, only to find a little tired old man.

There *was* bustling energy in Berlin while we were there, but it was coming from the West. As we ran, we could see dozens of construction cranes dominating the city skyline like mythic giants. Berlin was a city in transition, and as I ran the course, I thought it would be interesting to come back and race the city again in a few years to see what it would grow to be.

Everything about the Berlin Marathon was as I expected it to be, but after crossing the finish line, I encountered one of the oddest sights I'd yet seen at a race: race volunteers carrying large bundles of cash for on-the-spot deposit refunds for race chips. I couldn't imagine anyone flashing wads of cash like that in Central Park in New York City, not even on marathon day with mounted police nearby. Fuhgeddaboutit.

After Berlin, I ran the Marine Corps and New York marathons again—a personal tradition at this point—and then ended 1999 by adding Washington State and Florida to my list of completed states. That made it eleven marathons in 1999, which was a new record for me, and I had reached marathon number fifty, the halfway point in my quest. But I didn't stop to ponder it, because I was busy running marathons in South Carolina, Maryland, Boston again, and Maine. Next up: joining a running group to head to Beijing for marathon number 55.

Beijing, like Berlin, was another city in transition. Its biggest changes would not come until years later, when it began building up in earnest for 2008 Olympic Games, but even in October 2000 there were signs of the coming transformation. There were more cars than I expected to see, and the clothes and bicycles of the younger Chinese were flashier and more colorful than the dour, drab designs sported by their elders.

Our tour guide helped minimize communication problems, but there was still opportunity for misadventure. One day, with no group activity scheduled, another team member and I climbed into a taxi, aiming to visit a local temple. We showed a photo of our intended destination to the driver, then sat back in the cab. Before long, the driver turned onto a highway, and as the miles and minutes ticked by, my friend and I exchanged nervous glances. After a 45-minute odyssey, the cab pulled up in front of a marketplace. We had no idea where we were, but we knew one thing: if we let that cab drive away, we might never find our way back. Having had the foresight to bring a book of matches from our hotel, we showed it to the driver and pointed at the address. He shrugged, and set off to return us to where we started. We never did make it to that temple, but things could have turned out much worse.

On race day, my traveling companions and I gathered with the other runners in Tiananmen Square. As we waited for the start, I looked around and tried to imagine the confrontation a decade earlier between government troops and the mass of protesters who had camped there. Our group had talked about it, but it was a topic that none of the local Chinese seemed willing or able to discuss with us. On race day, there was no dissent visible among those gathered; we were all runners. Crossing the cultural divide, I bartered my American running jacket for a Chinese Olympic team jacket, a deal consummated wordlessly with a Chinese runner, using rough pantomime to transcend our language barrier. It's a marathon treasure that's as meaningful to me as many of the medals I've earned.

Finally, we all gathered at the start line, and the familiar crack of the starter's gun sent us out on a loop of the square, under the larger-than-life gaze of Chairman Mao. His stern image was everywhere—not only on official posters but also on clock faces, shirts, mugs, and souvenir trinkets. He seemed to be making a transition himself, from revered leader to high camp. Ironic comeuppance for a despot.

After exiting Tiananmen Square and racing through the city, we were herded out onto one of the city's surrounding highways, where we tallied most of the miles in our race. The few spectators we passed stood in hushed observance, offering support with only an occasional clap or shout. After the spectacular start, the rest of the race was, to be honest, a very boring slog.

We finished our race on the highway, an appropriate end to a mostly disappointing race. I was still glad to have to have made the journey, though, especially after visiting an unrestored section of the Great Wall in an area well outside of Beijing. Still, the race itself seemed like a missed opportunity for the Chinese. A marathon should be used as a forum to showcase a city, to give visitors a glimpse into its natural and architectural beauty, its history, and its culture. Beijing had so much to offer, and yet the race did so little with it.

In addition to running on foreign soil, I undertook another challenge that year; in addition to my regular job, I became a marathon coach for a charity fundraising team in my spare time. I had jumped from being a marathoner to being a marathon evangelist. In 2000, I signed on with the Arthritis Foundation's Joints in Motion program, and the following year also signed up to coach the American Diabetes Association's Team Diabetes. Coaching forced me to articulate many of my beliefs about marathoning, and also to reconsider the elements of my training regimen. It was a great way to share my passion for marathoning, and I grew to love it. Also, as the old Navy recruiting posters used to say, it was a great way to see the world. I traveled with these teams to Dublin, Rome, Athens, and Amsterdam, and in each of these places, I ran along with them. I was as happy as an obsessed runner could be; I was helping charities and sharing my love for the marathon as I experienced races all around the world.

The trade-off, however, was my commitment to never running a marathon all-out if I was with a team. I didn't want to be in a position where I might be unavailable to help my team, whether from injury or mental and physical fatigue. I wanted to be able to not only finish the marathon with the runners I was pacing, but to also run back and see after our other, slower participants.

Still, it was an enormously rewarding experience. Many of our team members had never considered themselves athletes, and by the end of our time together, they had discovered a strength and resolve they never knew they possessed. This realization was a powerful thing, and I was thrilled to be part of it for so many people.

My first trip abroad with a charity team was for the Dublin Marathon, in October 2000, just two weeks after Beijing. Conditions in Ireland were brutal that year, as race day greeted us with driving rain and high winds. During the race, I tried ducking behind larger runners to lessen the impact of the wind, like a cyclist drafting another rider. Nothing helped, though. It was just one of those days.

The Irish fans seemed undisturbed by bad weather, however. They lined the roads and shouted "Well done, lads!" to the runners flying past. One spectator in particular remains in my memory: at mile 11, a golden-haired girl, no more than seven or eight years old, looked up hopefully as we ran past and squealed, "Give us a smile!" Those of us within earshot of this little sprite couldn't help but comply.

One unexpected feature of the race was that rather than hand out cups of water like they do in the States, the race volunteers in Dublin handed out full bottles. Not a bad idea, except that few runners drank the entire bottle, or even carried it for very long. The result: for the block or two after each water stop, half-filled water bottles flew through the air like hand grenades.

At the finish line, exhausted, shivering runners were treated to coffee and chocolate—not the bananas and bagels found at most races, but still very welcome. It had been a grueling day. I felt worst for the first-time runners, who perhaps didn't know that a marathon didn't have to be this hard. They had conquered more than the usual marathon challenge, and I tried to help them realize that. They were finally convinced by the front page of *The Irish Times* the following morning, which ran the headline "Runners Defy Wind and Rain in Marathon of Suffering." I kept that page, and have it somewhere still, buried in a stack of race memorabilia.

One month later, I found myself flying out to Hawaii with a different charity team for the Honolulu Marathon. Although we were still technically in the United States, Hawaii felt exotic. Perhaps that was because Hawaii is the only state with an historic palace, and because so many Japanese runners had entered the marathon. At one store, I actually wondered for a moment if they accepted dollars, proving true the old saying, better to be silent and thought a fool, rather than speak and remove all doubt.

In most marathons, my plan is to start out comfortably and slowly ease into my goal race pace, saving enough energy in reserve for a fast finish. But in Honolulu, with the threat of a hot sun weighing heavily on me, I decided to flip my strategy; I would start out fast and try to get as many miles as possible under my belt before the heat set in. It was a risky strategy, especially since I was committed to keeping some energy in reserve to use helping my team afterward, but I felt sure the best strategy would be to do what I could to avoid running more than necessary in the hot tropical sun.

We were in the Christmas holiday season, but the weather was warm as we lined up with 20,000 other runners in the predawn darkness in Waikiki, awaiting the traditional fireworks show that accompanied the race start. After looping Waikiki, we were sent out for two loops around Diamondhead, the volcano that dominated the Honolulu waterfront skyline. Despite my attempts to avoid spending too much time in the sun, I still found myself feeling dehydrated and depleted by the time

I made it to the finish line in Kapiolani Park 3 hours and 25 minutes after having started the race. Luckily, I recovered quickly, and was able to head out back on the course to run with my team and make sure they were all having the experience they had trained so faithfully for. And as for me, marathon number 57 was in the books, and Hawaii was on my list of states.

Running Tip #8

Avoid Dehydration

Your body uses water, in the form of sweat, to shed heat. This water comes mostly from blood plasma, and unless you replace it, your heart won't be able to pump the resulting sludge to your working muscles. As little as a 2 percent loss in body fluid can seriously affect exercise performance. Loss of blood plasma also makes it harder for your heart to send blood to the skin to cool off your core. When this happens, you risk heat exhaustion, and even heat stroke, which can be fatal.[6]

Signs of dehydration

- *Dry skin*
- *Cold or clammy skin*
- *Nausea*
- *Disorientation*

---

6 There's been some research, especially by Dr. Timothy Noakes of the University of Cape Town—who himself has run more than seventy marathons and ultramarathons—suggesting that dehydration isn't really dangerous at all. Instead, he argues, it actually helped early man hunt game across the open plains by reducing his body weight. Rising core temperatures and reduced speed are not caused by dehydration, he says, but instead by overexertion. While these are certainly intriguing ideas, and might very well be true, I'd recommend caution here, and stick for the time being with the conservative viewpoint until more research is done in this area.

Your plan of attack

- *Drink regularly*. Water is the old standby, but a sports drink also replaces essential minerals and provides some simple sugars for fuel. Drinking is the key; what you drink is up to you.
- *Weigh yourself*. Comparing your weight before and after exercise will tell you how much fluid you need to replace under various conditions.
- *If in doubt, act*. Slow down and take in more fluids. Slurp water from a garden hose, or knock on someone's door and explain your problem. Pour cool water on your wrists, arms and head. Sit down in a shady area. If you don't feel better quickly, call 911. Don't be brave; this is a potentially dangerous situation.

Island Running

As the jet descended toward the runway, it wasn't hard for me to remember why I had decided to come to Bermuda. Looking out the window, I saw palm trees. It was the middle of January, 2001, and here I was, looking at *palm trees.* Back home in Washington, D.C., I wouldn't see green outdoors for another two months or so. The temperature, as promised in the Department of Tourism brochures, was in the mid-60s, with cloudy skies. A little warm for running, perhaps, but I knew what to do about that, right?

Often thought of as one of the Caribbean islands, Bermuda actually lies far to the north, some 570 miles east of the North Carolina coast. Although it's commonly considered a single island, it is actually a collection of some 150 separate islands, many of them no more than a speck of rock peeking above the bright blue waters. They are the tips of long-dormant volcanoes, together forming a long, fishhook-shaped archipelago, inhabited by some 61,000 people. Because these islands are swept by the friendly Gulf Stream winds, the temperature in Bermuda stays moderate all year long, with temperatures ranging from a low in the upper 60 degrees Fahrenheit, to a high in the mid-to-upper 70 degrees Fahrenheit.

In the middle of this fishhook is the city of Hamilton, established in 1790 as a convenient meeting place for all of Bermuda's scattered residents. Now the capital of Bermuda, its streets are filled with pubs, restaurants, and little shops. The main thoroughfare here is Front Street, which runs parallel to the harbor, and which features a roofed sentry box affectionately called "the birdcage," from which a police officer directs traffic.

Near the birdcage on Front Street is the Number 1 Passenger Terminal, site of the race packet pick-up. When I arrived to get my number, I found that the field would be, well, an *intimate* gathering of runners. There were only 392 runners registered for the full marathon, and 313 registered for the half. This was a far cry from the huge crowds at the marathons in New York, Boston, and Chicago, but small races do have their charm.

I spent the rest of the day doing a little sightseeing and a little eating, but mostly just resting and waiting. Rain was predicted, and sure enough, I heard the tapping of rain splashing against the window in the middle of the night. By the time I got up and went out the door, though, the rain had tapered off, leaving a cool, overcast morning. Perfect.

By 8 A.M., I was back on Front Street for the start of the race. The course is a double loop, with the half-marathoners pulling over to the side in Hamilton as the marathoners forge ahead for another lap.

I always have mixed feeling about that kind of format. It's nice to muster the entire running crowd together for as long as possible, especially in small races, but it's also quite a letdown to head toward the half-marathoner finish line with a pack of runners, and emerge alone on the other side.

As the starter's gun went off and we surged up Front Street, I thought about The Hill. When I first began to consider running the Bermuda Marathon, my first question was, where's the hill? In a marathon, there's almost *always* a hill. Sure enough, it's there: a nearly 40-meter climb at 3½ miles called McGall's Hill, revisited at 16½ miles.

The first mile flashed by in a blur of storefronts and adrenaline, and then we slipped out of the city center, onto a beautiful country road heading east. The road wasn't crowded, but neither was it empty; there were runners everywhere. We rolled over a few small rises, and then we were upon The Hill. It looked impressive, but it was early in the race, and we collectively ate it up.

Green. I'd noticed it upon arriving, but now I saw it everywhere. Lush green, bright green. The island doesn't have a soil base deep and rich enough to support large-scale agriculture, but its native plants thrive tenaciously, lining the marathon course with color. And there were other colors as well: houses splashed with blues and yellows and pinks, with bright white rooftops, kept clean so rainwater falling from their sides may be captured in underground cisterns for later use.

I noticed something else, too. Something that was *not* there. Garbage. I didn't see any trash along the streets, not in Hamilton, not on the country roads, not anywhere. So far, it was a runners' paradise.

We turned north onto the wonderfully-named Devil's Hole Road, and soon, at mile five, we were treated to a spectacular view of Harrington Sound. From there we turned toward Flatts Village, a former smugglers' haven that served as the site for the execution of witches in the mid-1600s. Today, the village is a benign and friendly haven for sailboats and fishermen, and true to its name, it was flat. The crowds had been sparse so far, but now there were several small groups of spectators. They seemed interested and supportive, though more reserved than the usual marathon crowd. That didn't surprise me. Bermuda, as a British possession, retains some Old World mannerisms that were brought across the Pond, including a tradition of high tea. Bermudans don't scream and yell along the course, but they are quick to return a polite "hello" or "good morning."

After Flatts Village, we turned onto North Shore Road. It was here, at mile 8, that I was rewarded with the first ocean view of the race, and it was breathtaking. Jagged dark volcanic rock met glorious blue water in a spray of white foam. It was almost enough to make me stop to enjoy the moment, but I knew I'd be back to see it again on my second loop.

The road settled into a pattern of rolling hills, and I noticed that the porous limestone, used widely as a building material, left structures appearing weathered and ancient. A stone archway overhead looked absolutely medieval. I also noticed the salty breeze blowing in off the ocean—another welcome distraction. On the left were signs for the Railway Trail, a running path made up of segments from Bermuda's old narrow gauge railway line, completed in 1931 and abandoned in 1947. It looked full of beauty and adventure, carved through rock and draped in foliage. I fought the urge to veer off and explore it. At mile 11 we turned south, back toward Hamilton. An old man sitting in a folding chair by the side of the road called out, "Once you pass me, it's easy to the finish!" I called back, "See you again soon!" I hoped I would.

The last 2 miles into Hamilton were downhill and fast. The sun fought its way through the clouds and scattered them, and the foliage retreated. The temperature climbed as the halfway point loomed ahead and the half-marathoners put on a burst of speed. I joined them and flew through the finish line, but my race was only half over, and my legs suddenly seemed to lose their bounce. McGall's Hill, redux, was just 3 miles away. As I tried to regain my focus and marshal my reserves, a man on a scooter passed by and offered me a candy. "I'll be with you guys all the way!" he promised as he sped ahead to the next runner. An older Japanese man passed me and called out "I'm faster than last year!" "Good for you!" I yelled back, and felt energized by his enthusiasm. I threw an invisible lasso around him, and let him pull me along for a few miles. Before long, I found my stride again, and settled into a groove.

And just in time, too. McGall's Hill loomed ahead, and it seemed to have grown since I'd last seen it. That leaden feeling crept back into my legs, and I concentrated on just moving ahead, putting one foot in front of the next. Looking off to my left I saw rolling green fields. Sitting there on the hillside was a woman with long brown hair, with her dog by her side. She smiled and waved, and I waved back.

And then I was at the top of the hill. This time, I noticed that there was a church on the hilltop, and, to its right, a cemetery. I was glad I didn't notice it earlier; it would have seemed too ominous. But not now; McGall's Hill was history.

Now I relaxed, remembering the flat miles that lay ahead. The heat was taking its toll, however, and I worried that soon I would start slowing down. As I re-entered Flatts Village, I tried to put a confident face on my running, for myself as well as for the spectators. I heard someone call out "You're seventeenth!" Me? Really? I've never had someone yell out my place during a race before. One more benefit of a small race field. It was enough to give me a boost over the next few miles.

I realized that the crowds, sparse though they were, were as determined as the runners to see the race through. They remembered me from my first lap, and called out as I passed by. The children waved and the women smiled. "You're looking good!" the old women said. "You too!" I replied, and they laughed and laughed. The old man I saw on the first loop, still sitting in his chair, waved to me like he's known me for years, and up ahead I saw Runner Number 16. It seemed that he wasn't that far ahead.

The street signs read "4 kilometers to Hamilton," and I tried to accelerate. The scooter-man pulled alongside again. No thanks, no candy for me, but thank you, thank you. More people lined the path now, and I started counting down the minutes I thought I had left to run. Mile 25 was downhill, and I wondered whether the extra speed I gained from the descent was worth the pain in my legs and lungs. But there was Mr. 16, and I was near to him, very near, then next to him. He smiled and said hello. I smiled back, and surged onward. Up ahead was Front Street again, and the finish line, meant for me this time. I crossed it, relieved and grateful for having completed another marathon, to have another medal. I turned around, and there was Mr. 16th, though now he was 17th. We smiled, less competitors now than comrades-in-arms.

I stepped inside the terminal, and went upstairs where there was the promise of food and drink. I took in fluids during the race, but it was so hot, and now I was so thirsty. Race Secretary Pam Shailer told me that it actually *hailed* during race weekend the previous year, and I was happy to have been spared any rain or ice. There were pastries, fruit, hot chocolate, and soup laid out for us, and soon I felt revived. Downstairs, there were two massage therapists ministering to the runners, and I got in line. When it was my turn, the therapist introduced himself—his name was John Ford, and he seemed to know just about everyone there. More importantly, his fingers were magic, and brought welcome relief to my tired body.

Marathon number 58 was in the books.

Running Tip #9

Avoid Hyponatremia

Hyponatremia is the opposite of dehydration; it's a dilution of sodium and other electrolytes caused by drinking too much water, which is most common among athletes who are on the marathon course for more than 4½ hours. It can be deadlier than dehydration, and in extreme cases, can lead to coma or even death.

Because its symptoms are similar to those of dehydration, hyponatremia is often misdiagnosed. The first question to ask a runner in distress is how much water have they been drinking? That will tell you what their problem likely is.

Over-the-counter nonsteroidal anti-inflammatory drugs ("NSAIDs"), such as aspirin, naproxen sodium (Aleve), and ibuprofen (Advil and Motrin), seem to increase the risk, perhaps because they inhibit the body's ability to excrete water. Women might also be at higher risk because they're smaller than men and can more easily overload on water.

Symptoms

- *fatigue*
- *cramping*
- *dizziness, nausea and vomiting*
- *bloating and puffiness in the face and fingers*
- *headache, confusion, and fainting*

Prevention

- *Use sports drinks that contain sodium.*

- *Add salt to your food in hot weather, unless you're on a salt-restricted diet.*

- *If you feel symptoms of hyponatremia while running, eat some salty food, like pretzels.*

- *Don't take any NSAIDs immediately before or during your race; if you must take a pain reliever, take acetaminophen (Tylenol).*

Running Here, Running There, Running Everywhere!

In March 2001, I traveled with an American Diabetes Association fund-raising team to Italy for the Rome Marathon. With the ancient Coliseum as a backdrop, the race start was as impressive a sight as one could ever hope to find. As I stood shoulder to shoulder with the mass of other runners, I realized that I'd never before encountered such a stink from a race crowd, particularly before the event even started. Did no one here ever use deodorant?

Self-preservation led me to work my way out of the crush in search of fresh air. I wriggled to the outside, and wandered forward, where the elite runners waited in secure corrals. I saw the Africans, loose and smiling and confident. And there was an Italian team, laughing, standing around ... and smoking. I blinked in disbelief. Yep, there they were, sneaking in a last butt before the gun went off. *Only in Italy*, I thought.

With the race start just minutes away, I gulped in a lungful of fresh air and dove back into the crowd. Suddenly the mass surged forward. I assumed that the race staff had opened up the corrals, and that the crowd was pressing forward toward the starting line. I expected that our advance would soon grind to a halt, but somehow the crowd kept pressing forward. Soon there was enough room for us to break into an easy run. I couldn't understand what was going on.

Slowly it dawned on me that the race had begun. There had been no announcement, no starting gun, and no countdown. The race utilized an electronic chip system, to track each runner, but still, it was a very unsettling way to start a race. A friend with more European racing experience than I had later told me that this was typical of races abroad; if the runners get impatient, the officials just send them, like a mother telling her whining kids, *Fine, you want to go out and play so badly, well, go!*

Organization continued to be a problem after the race was under way. The first water stop wasn't ready for us by the time we came streaking by. Since Rome, like many European marathons, provide water and sports drinks every 5 kilometers—3.1 miles to us Americans—rather than the traditional mile or two in the United States, that meant that many runners went without any water for the first 6 miles of the race. It was already shaping up to be a hot, sunny day, so I knew that dehydration would be a problem. I began forcing down extra fluids as soon as drinks were available, and I told the runners I was pacing to do the same.

Not everyone was thinking ahead, though. I spotted a runner from the Canadian Diabetes Association, who was wearing an outrageous sunburst team singlet, in contrast to the solid red shirt that my Team Diabetes runners wore. I introduced myself. His name was Geoff, and he was running his first marathon. I was pacing several of my teammates already, and we all decided to run together. Geoff was running very well, but he hadn't been taking in enough fluids, and as the miles wore on he began to cramp. My teammates and I made sure he drank more, helped him stretch, and even rubbed his aching calves. Geoff urged us to go on, but I told him that if I surged ahead to the finish line, this would be just another race for me, neither the best nor the worst of my finishing times. But if I stayed with him and made sure he finished, it would make the race much more meaningful. The other runners in our little group agreed, and we decided to finish the race together.

We continued past the Vatican and the Circus Maximus, down cobblestone streets and narrow alleys. The cobblestones turned out to be more foe than friend, as they robbed our legs of their bounce and left them sore and aching. Spectators yelled out *forza!* (strength). At one point I overheard a spectator yell out *bocca al lupo!* as we passed, to which one of my runners yelled back *crepi il lupo!* I asked the runner what all that ruckus was about.

"Ah," he said, "that's just something people say in Italy during races. He yelled, 'you're in the mouth of the wolf!' and I called back the traditional response, 'may the wolf die!' It's how they wish you good luck." Like almost everything Italian, it was more dramatic than how things are done back home.

As we ran, we picked up a few more Team Diabetes runners who were happy to share in the team spirit. Finally, the Coliseum, and the finish line, loomed up ahead. We crossed the finish line and celebrated like it was New Year's Eve. It was as happy a finish as I've ever seen, and Geoff thanked me by giving me his team singlet—more appreciated once I'd laundered it!—as well as buying me several beers at our team get-together that evening. The friendship we forged proved to be lasting; Geoff and I kept in touch after we returned home, updating each other on our lives and running, keeping alive the hope that we'll be able to meet up for another marathon someday.

After returning from Rome, I ran Boston again—I was becoming a regular, though I never took it for granted—and then I met up with Dave in Austria for the Vienna Marathon in May. He was there for work, and the timing seemed too good to pass up. We raced along the Danube, passing beautiful parks and buildings, as the Viennese called out "*Hopp hopp!*" meaning, "jump faster!" I felt like I was where I was supposed to be, doing what I was supposed to be doing. I was flying around the world, meeting wonderful people, running marathons, and also feeling like I was making a difference in people's lives. It all felt like an amazing dream. Everything was perfect.

It was May of 2001. It was the last season of our national innocence, before everything would change forever.

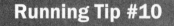

Running Tip #10

Travel Like a Runner

Before you go

- *Be willing to go it alone.* It's more fun to travel with friends, but you can make new friends easily during a race.
- *Clip your toenails before you leave home.* That's one less thing to worry about, and one less piece of equipment to risk getting confiscated by security.
- *Bring only carry-on baggage.* You'll be able to safeguard your racing gear, and you can more easily switch flights if there are any delays, or take advantage of requests for volunteers to give up their seats in exchange for free-flight vouchers.
- *Make a list of the essentials, and pack before the day of departure.* But don't panic if you forget something; unless you're traveling to a remote locale, you can still buy what you need when you arrive.

Be prepared for the flight

- *Drink plenty of water and bring your own healthy snacks.* Bring your own bottle and ask flight attendants to fill it.
- *Flex your legs or move around often.* The risk of developing potentially life-threatening blood clots during a long flight is higher among runners, perhaps because of our lower heart rate and blood pressure. Wearing compression socks might also help.

Have a plan

- *Deal with time zone changes.* Plan on one day of adjustment for every hour you lost or gained, although sometimes not adjusting works better if you're traveling east to west and you have a very early race start.
- *Scout around.* Become familiar with the course and the city. If you're racing in a high altitude, arrive in town a week early, or add 30 seconds per mile to your expected race pace.

Speed Dreams

It was a conundrum. I loved marathons so much that I wanted to run them as often as possible, yet the more I ran them, the harder it would be for me to reach my potential as a marathoner. Running a marathon just about every month relieved me of the need to do long training runs, since my races *were* my long training runs. But I sacrificed intense training between races, since I was usually either recovering from one race or tapering for the next. I knew that I was also preventing my body from fully recovering from each of my marathon efforts. This hadn't resulted in injury, but I wasn't priming my body for one supreme effort, the one that would get me to my next goal in running: a sub-three hour marathon.

Finally, in the summer of 2001, I decided to take up the challenge. I had run six marathons in the first half of the year, but I committed to making my next one—number 64—"The One." I took a month off from hard running to let my body fully rest, then picked the Steamtown Marathon in Scranton, Pennsylvania, in October as my target race. My work colleague and running buddy Jim was planning on doing it, and had been talking up its virtues. It was known as a fast race, mostly downhill, with a net drop of 955 feet. Eventually I was won over, and signed up, hoping that as long as I could keep my feet moving, I could count on gravity to bring me home in record time

That summer, Jim and I trained ferociously. Although I had done speed work with my running friends and run marathons with them, I had never before focused on a single race with any of them. Jim and I developed a unique camaraderie, stopping by each other's office with updates on our workouts and pace calculations. Our lunchtime tempo sessions, run faster than race pace, were epic. I loved them, and began to keep a journal to record my thoughts.

It's Thursday afternoon, and Jim is waiting for me. Today is our tempo run, a 10-mile loop that is supposed to leave us breathless and exhilarated. Last week Jim ran strong, and opened a half-block lead over me with two miles left. I forced my leaden legs to give just a little bit more, and Jim slowed just a bit to let me pull even. Afterward, I was exhausted. And now Jim is waiting for me again.

We start out easy, weaving through crowds and traffic. The D.C. parks insinuate themselves through the city like vines wrapping around a tree. Our loop takes us from the downtown business district to Georgetown, and from there onto a 3-mile wooded trail. We would emerge at the northern edge of the city and run down Connecticut Avenue, back to our starting point. It's a beautiful route, about 10 miles long, but it's also our proving ground. These weekly runs are an important part of my plan to build speed for Steamtown. If I can just keep up with Jim.

We work our way through Georgetown, and enter the woods. We're running well, but shorter on breath than either of us would like. Our conversation dwindles down to a few short words, and then just the sound of our heavy breathing. As we jump logs and hop over streambeds, I imagine that I'm an early settler, chasing game for the family dinner. Or perhaps an escaped convict, with the howl of bloodhounds getting ever louder behind me. Leaves brush past my face, and I feel a surge of energy. I pick up the pace.

We leave the woods, and I glance down at my watch. We're ahead of our usual pace, but the toughest part lies ahead. The downhill must be run hard if it is to be run honestly. It's a 4-mile stretch that should leave my lungs burning and my thoughts muddled. Less effort than that makes it just another easy run, and puts Jim a half block ahead of me.

We sweep down the avenue and overtake a bus picking up passengers. I consider the traffic lights ahead, and the scheduled stops the bus has to make. We'll run along the bus route for the next three miles, and if we run hard, I think to myself, we can beat it. Again, I pick up the pace.

Now we're flying, our bodies moving smoothly, feet barely touching the ground. We've raced the bus a full mile, and it still hasn't gotten the better of us. It pulls close, flirts with us, but then brakes to pick up passengers, or is halted by a red light. I become accustomed to the ebb and flow of its loud, droning engine. And then the National Zoo appears, its entrance gate enveloped by a swarm of tourists. We step out toward the street, and collect the open-mouthed stares of children. I pick up the pace.

Ahead is the bridge over Rock Creek Park. This is where I watched Jim surge ahead last week and was unable to match his strength. Today, my lungs are burning, but I feel strong. Jim falls a few strides behind, surges to make up lost ground, then falls back and surges again. He will not gain a half block on me today. The bus is behind us now for good, vanquished. We have less than two miles to go. I pick up the pace.

Now we make a left onto broad Massachusetts Avenue for the last few blocks of our run. We are running without thinking, like machines, just trying to hold on. "Almost there, just a little bit more," I intone, as much for myself as for Jim. And then we are just one block away. I am tired, but I am in love with the effort, and I tell Jim I will sprint the last block. He joins me, and we tear down the street, mad for speed and adrenaline.

And then the workout is over. We shuffle, letting our heartbeats slow and our breathing return to normal. I look at my watch. Six minutes faster than last week. "Great run," Jim says breathlessly. "Great run. My best 10-miler ever." I smile and nod, happy and alive.

We take turns, Jim and I, pulling and pushing each other through our training runs, tearing through the woods and racing buses, chasing after our marathon dreams. We are athletes in the greatest, craziest, most competitive, most supportive, most elegant, most brutal sport in the world. And next week, with any luck, Jim will be waiting for me again, ready to hit the trails.

That was my summer: sweat and effort and dirty running clothes. The days shortened, and a chill crept into the air, and summer faded behind us.

It was September, 2001.

When I was growing up, my parents and my older relatives would sometimes recall exactly where they were and what they were doing when President Kennedy had been shot. It seemed so odd to me for so many people to have such a personal memory of such a famous moment.

Not any more.

I recall exactly where I was and what I was doing on the morning of September 11th. I was in a neighborhood local gym where I trained, making my way through a cardio session on some of the cross-training machines. I distracted myself by looking up at the overhead TVs, catching the morning news. Little by little, reports came in about an errant plane that had struck one of the World Trade Center towers. Like everyone else, I thought it must have been an accident, similar to when a plane struck the Empire State Building decades before. But of course, it was nothing like that, and as the events of that morning unfolded, I stayed glued to my LifeCycle, extending my workout from one hour, to two, to three. I couldn't leave my seat, and almost compulsively, maniacally, I kept pedaling.

Reports of the second plane hitting a tower came in, and the footage was horrible and mesmerizing. At one point, as the commentators talked on about what was happening in Manhattan, I realized the footage of a smoking building being shown on TV wasn't the World Trade Center; it was the Pentagon, right here in my city's backyard. Obviously, something had happened there as well, but hadn't yet been reported. I climbed down from the exercise bike. Everything seemed unreal as I made my way downstairs. By the time I got there, a staff member at the front desk told me that one of the towers had collapsed. The second one followed shortly after.

I called my office and spoke to one of my friends there. He told me that everyone who was there was preparing to leave, and that I shouldn't bother coming in. I cleaned up and went over to visit a friend who lived on the top floor of an apartment building. He had a beautiful view of the city, facing south to the Potomac River. Toward the Pentagon.

When I arrived there, I found that several others had come as well. We stared at the horizon, where a smoke cloud hung in the air. It was the first tangible proof that something terrible had happened. We sat most of the day with our eyes glued to the television, taking in the reports and trying to make sense of it all.

The next meeting of my charity marathon training group was somber. Instead of being upbeat and boisterous as usual, they were quiet and apprehensive. We had been training for a return trip to the Dublin Marathon, but with our departure only a month and a half away, there was little chance that we would see a return to normalcy before we were scheduled to depart. This was what we had to deal with.

We started off by talking about the toll that the recent events had taken on all of us. I said that I planned to continue training the group and would go to Dublin, as I hoped all of them would also do. Some people said that they no longer felt comfortable leaving the country. I wanted to tell them that everything would be okay and that they should still go, but how could anyone be sure?

Most of the runners opted to continue with the program. We would continue training, and go to Dublin. I hoped that I had not just put all of their lives at risk.

Meanwhile, Jim and I made it through our own training program, and drove out to Scranton on October 6, the day before the Steamtown Marathon. Scranton is an old locomotive town, and though its glory years are long gone, it honors its past with a museum and, of course, the race. I had calculated that I needed to run at a 6:51-per-mile pace to get my sub-3-hour time. 6:51. Just thinking about those numbers made me nervous.

On race day I felt good. The skies were clear, and there was a slight chill in the air. I did a light warm-up, and waited for the starter's gun, shaking my legs, looking for clues as to how they felt. Did they feel strong? Did they have pop? Was I hungry? Stuffed? Thirsty? Bloated? I considered it all, and decided everything was right. I was ready to go.

The race started, and we ran through the city streets, immediately lurching downhill. I was breathing cleanly, strongly. We twisted and turned on the city streets, and soon left them behind, heading out toward quieter roads. I felt great. I pulled ahead of Jim and weaved through the small crowd, feeling like I was hardly touching the ground. As we ran past tall trees bathed in green leaves, I struck up a conversation with a man next to me, and then passed him behind. I had never felt so good before so early in a race. I pitied all the other animals in nature for their slowness. I looked down at my watch. I was running 20–30 seconds faster than my goal pace. I should have been worried; energy is like a bank account, and if you spend it in one place, particularly early in a race, it won't be there later when you really need it. I was blowing my reserves with wild abandon, but I felt confident that I was fine. I had trained hard, and this was the pace that felt comfortable. Perhaps my energy account had accrued interest, I thought. I would not slow down. I would run hard and hold on to the finish line. It would be like Boston, but better.

It wouldn't take long for me to realize how wrong I was. I had carefully drawn up a training plan and spent months following it, but then I threw all that hard work away on race day. It was a rookie mistake, and there's a price to be paid for such recklessness. By mile 16, I knew that I would have to ante up. I hadn't yet slowed, but that intoxicating energy was ebbing, and I realized that I wouldn't be able to sustain the pace I had set. If I could just keep running well, though, I told myself, I still could make my sub-3-hour goal.

Over the next few miles, I slowly began to accept the reality of my situation. The hard downhill running had taken a toll on my quadriceps. I began to consider fallback goals as my sub-3-hour dream began to slip away. By mile 20 I was running on a beautiful bicycle path through the woods, but I couldn't enjoy it. I was in trouble, and like a beaten fighter looking for a place to fall down, I began to consider when I would start walking.

Walk breaks are an accepted part of racing for many people, especially first-time marathoners, and I recommend them to my teams. When you take a walk break, you give your running muscles a moment's rest, and you also give your mind a manageable goal to work with: just run reasonably hard for another mile, and then you can have another walk break. Breaking the race up into segments like that makes it seem much easier to handle. As I've told my teams, the marathon is just too big to swallow in one gulp.

In Steamtown, though, my walk breaks during the last 6 miles of the race were not strategic. They were acts of desperation. My legs ached with fatigue, and they demanded that I stop running. As soon as I started walking, the race I had trained for was effectively over. I managed to talk my legs into running again for a few minutes at a time over the final few miles, but as the minutes ticked by, I saw even my various fallback goals slip away. First, my dream of a sub-3 hour finish vanished, followed shortly by my hopes for a new personal record. Eventually, I realized that I would not even achieve a Boston qualifying time. Finally, I reached the last stop on my descent: I just wanted to finish the race. When it was finally, mercifully, over, my official time was 3:20:14. Not bad, really: it was the eighth best time of the sixty-four marathons I had run, but that was a deceiving statistic. The Steamtown Marathon had broken me.

As I gathered myself and waited for Jim, I thought about a story a childhood friend recently told me. Supposedly, a new guy had recently walked into a gym back in New York where we used to train and started boasting about how much he could lift. "It's all mind over matter," he said. "If I can believe it, my body can achieve it." With that, he loaded 300 pounds onto the bench press, laid down on the bench, lifted the bar off the support, and ... crashed it down onto his face, knocking out three teeth.

The lesson, of course, is that mind over matter works *as long as you're in the ballpark*. I could believe with all my heart and soul that I could fly, but if I jump out of a top floor window, I'm still going to go splat on the sidewalk.

That's how I felt about my performance in Steamtown. I went splat. There was nothing in my training to justify the early pace I had set for myself. My training hadn't put me in the ballpark for the race I was running. It was a difficult lesson to learn, especially at this late date, when I already had a dozen years of marathoning experience behind me and should have known better. As much as I tried to put on a happy face, it was hard for me to hide my sadness and anger. I had wasted a good opportunity to achieve something special.

Once, long ago, I swore to myself that if ever I crossed a marathon finish line and was disappointed, I would hang up my running shoes. Was it now time for me to quit? I thought things over during the long drive home. By the time I reached my apartment, I had reconciled myself to what had happened. I decided that whatever my original goal had been, finishing the race was still a wonderful achievement, especially given how badly I felt during those last few miles. I could have quit, but didn't, and that was still something to be proud of.

I wasn't ready to hang up those shoes just yet.

Running Tip #11

Training Food

People exercising for 90 minutes should take in 4 calories per minute to maintain performance—that's up to 240 calories per hour. Not an easy task.

That's where sports gels come in. Basically, they are just sugary syrups, often caffeinated, that are easily digested for a quick mid-run energy boost.

- *Take with water.* They need water to break down, so take with 6–8 ounces of water. Sports drinks won't do the trick, since those extra carbs may be more than the stomach could absorb.
- *Experiment with the different flavors.*
- *Aim to take one every 45 minutes to an hour.*
- *Consider alternatives.* If you can't tolerate sports gels, experiment with other low-fat, easily-digested foods, like energy bars. There are even chewy bite-sized blocks and jelly beans especially for athletes.

Back to Where It All Began

I was glad to have worked my way through my disappointment with Steamtown so quickly, because my charity teams were making their final preparations for their own races. It wouldn't have helped them much to have a despondent coach.

First up was a return trip to Dublin. I was thrilled to be back; Dublin had become one of my favorite cities, and this time I knew exactly where I wanted to go and what I wanted to do. There was my favorite fish and chips stand next to the Jury's Hotel, and a pub in the Temple Bar district that had the best traditional Irish music. I also wanted to visit a great sweater shop I discovered on the previous trip, and revisit the beautiful Book of Kells at Trinity College.

And then, of course, there was also the race. This time we got lucky with the weather; skies were gray, but there was none of the rain and wind that had vexed us all the year before. All team members crossed the finish line without any significant problems, making me a happy coach indeed.

After the race was over, I set out with a woman I was dating and a few other people for a side trip to western Ireland, to visit Galway and the surrounding areas. The Irish countryside is starkly beautiful, with a checkerboard of stone fencing surrounding small, romantically weathered castles. We visited the Cliffs of Mohr, with its sudden and dramatic 700-foot drop. I was brave and cocky until we neared the cliff's edge, and then I chickened out like all the other visitors and got down on my belly and crawled to the edge to peer over the side.

I also learned the origin of the intricate piping patterns on the traditional Irish sweaters that I had bought. Traditionally, each clan was known by a particular pattern knit into their sweaters, much like a heraldic coat of arms. But instead of just being for show or vanity, these patterns served a grim purpose—they enabled the quick identification of drowned fisherman when their bodies were recovered. This was a harsh reminder that for all the beauty of the land, this could be a difficult and unforgiving place to live.

My Ireland trip drew to a close, but I wasn't ready to go home. I was about to meet up with another of my charity teams for a different adventure. We were going to visit the roots of the marathon, to retrace the steps taken by the ancients. We were going to Greece to run the Athens Marathon.

The racecourse would roughly follow the original route Phidippides supposedly traveled, from the still open and wind swept plains of Marathon, around the burial mound underneath which lay the remains of soldiers who fought that battle so long ago. From there, the route passed through the Greek countryside from town to town, until it reached its finish in the heart of Athens. It felt like a homecoming of sorts to me, though I'd never been there before. It was a race that I'd known for a long time that I would have to run.

Although cloaked in myth and legend, this event was still an actual race, and organizers would have to overcome the usual logistical problems. For years, the knock against the Athens Marathon was that it failed to provide enough water on the course. In 2001, the organizers finally solved that problem, placing drinks every 5 kilometers, and adding a few more water stops for good measure.

But we also had some unexpected water; the torrential downpour we missed in Ireland caught up with us in Greece. Most runners sought shelter in a nearby stadium construction site. Eventually, with clenched teeth and muttered curses, we all made our way through the downpour to the starting line. The race I had dreamed about for years was about to begin.

Running in the rain is not really such a bad experience. Even if it wasn't raining, we would all be soaked eventually by our own sweat. Our concern was really for our feet. When socks get wet, there's a greater chance of getting blisters, and a bad blister could ruin the most well-prepared athlete.

That day, things were not looking so good for our feet. Several sections of road were flooded under several feet of water. Some runners tried to cope by using garbage bags as waders, but discovered that the bags quickly tore and let water in. Others charged through, and either soaked their shoes or had them sucked off their feet by the thick mud below. Most of us just circled as wide as possible around these little lakes, climbing around grass and bushes. In the end, it didn't matter what each of us did; we were all going to get drenched by race's end. I was as soaked as I'd ever been, and that includes swimming.

The race presented other surprises as well. Athens is famous for its pack of wild, though mostly friendly, dogs. I had seen them and been trailed by them throughout the city, but I didn't expect to see them on race day. But there they were on the course, eyeing us curiously. Several of them decided to run alongside us for several kilometers. I was leery at first—even a friendly dog may be tempted to bite a runner—but they were as amiable and uncomplaining as any companion I've ever run with, and I was a bit sad when they decided not to go all the way with me to the finish line. They made a much better impression than the famous cats of Rome, who were nowhere to be found on race day.

Finally, the rain tailed off as we neared the outskirts of Athens. The traffic thickened, and stores and stop lights appeared. Near the 18-mile mark, we hit the big hill—there's always a big hill, remember?—and then we descended into the city for one of the most glorious finishes in marathoning: a loop on the track in the 1896 marble stadium that hosted the first modern Olympic Games. As the stadium came into view, my pulse quickened, and I picked up the pace for a strong finish. The course brought us closer to the stadium, and then ... led us past it. We had to run a little farther down the street and double back to the stadium. I felt like one of my canine companions might feel if a juicy steak waved in front of his nose, only to have it yanked away at the last second. It was a deflating moment, but when I finally did enter the stadium minutes later, my loop on that historic track made up for all the difficulties I'd had to overcome that day. It was my 66th marathon finish, and it was as sweet a moment as I'd ever had in road racing.

Running Tip #12

Running Etiquette

- *Stay to the right.* It's the rule with cars, and it should be the rule with people, too. Let faster runners and cyclists pass.
- *Don't run more than two people across.* If you hog the road, you're asking for trouble.
- *If you need to slow down or stop, step to the side.*
- *Be responsible for your own needs.* If you see someone else's cache of water or goodies sitting by the side of the road, don't touch it. They'll be counting on it being there when they need it. Choose training routes that pass by water fountains or convenience stores, or plant your own provisions by the side of road.
- *Be an honest racer.* If you're not a 5:30 mile, don't line up in the front of the pack before a race; you'll only get in the way of the faster runners. Plus, it's no fun getting passed.
- *Go the extra mile.* We're all part of a fitness community, and we should act like it. Wave and say hi to other runners, and offer extra water or goodies if you have them handy and someone looks like they could really use it. But be respectful of others; friendliness in the running community is not an invitation to distract or harass other runners.

As my marathon tally rose, I never gave up trying to understand my passion for the marathon. I knew instinctively that my running was meaningful in a way that I hadn't yet been able to explain, but now that I was recruiting and training team participants for my charity fund-raising teams, I knew that I had to find a way to articulate my reason for running 26.2 miles.

Information meetings usually began in the evening, after I had left my regular day job and my work as a lawyer. I began with the easy stuff, speaking about the joy of experiencing your body moving easily and powerfully, of the need to break through assumed or self-imposed limitations to discover the true potential hidden within all of us. I spoke of the satisfaction found in accomplishing the seemingly impossible, of proving wrong all those people who doubted not that it could be done, but that *they* could do it. I told them of my belief that everyone ought to have something they do that causes them to lose track of time, whether it's music or art or reading. For me, it's running. I rely on that quiet time to balance out the other demands on my life. I told them it might be the same for them as well.

Warmed up, I then spoke of the rewards to be found in accomplishing a difficult task. In a high school mythology class, we had been assigned Joseph Campbell's *The Hero with a Thousand Faces*, which explains the common threads of humankind's hero legends. The hero, Campbell explained, always sets out on a quest, separating himself from the ordinary routines of everyday life, and ventures to a land of danger. He confronts a great challenge, and after emerging triumphant, he returns home with a boon for mankind, whether fire, the Golden Fleece, defeat of the Minotaur, or great wisdom.

That is the hero's tale, I told my audience, and that is the tale of the marathoner, because the marathon is a heroic journey. Setting ourselves apart from our neighbors through our months-long ritual of training and sacrifice, we face the challenge of race day, when we test our resolve and preparation over miles of arduous roads, emerging, we hope, at the finish line, having gained wisdom about ourselves. Upon crossing that line, we are all of us transformed, having sensed our own power and determination, capable now of being masters of our fate rather than passive spectators.

I told them how running seems to bring out the best in all of us. I told them about Grete Waitz, the nine-time winner of the New York City Marathon. In 1993, Grete was in New York just as a friend of the race, and to support her husband, who was running. While she was there, she met Zoe Koplowitz, a marathoner who suffers from multiple sclerosis, and who competes while using crutches. It usually takes Zoe about 24 hours to finish a marathon, by which time there is hardly anyone at the finish line. Grete promised Zoe that she would wait for her at the finish line.

In the early hours of the morning following the race, Grete ran out to the finish line to see if Zoe was there yet; Zoe was close, but hadn't yet come into view. Then Grete discovered that there weren't any more finishers' medals left. Horrified and embarrassed, she ran back to her hotel room and grabbed her husband's medal, telling him "you don't really need another one," and made it back to the finish line in time to put it around Zoe's neck when she crossed it.

I told them that I often think of that story, about the caring of an elite runner for all the other brave people who attempt the marathon, and of the courage of a challenged runner like Zoe Koplowitz, whose achievement makes me thankful for simply having the opportunity to train and race. I don't know if running attracts good people, or if running makes people good, but there is a shared sense of understanding and respect among marathoners, a camaraderie forged by sweat and effort and sacrifice.

This is the marathon experience, I told them, and it is wondrous. I recalled for them the running of the 100th Boston Marathon in 1996, when defending champion Uta Pippig faded back behind young and strong Tegla Loroupe. It soon became apparent that Uta's difficulties were caused by the onset of menstruation and related intestinal problems, but Uta would not give in to the pain and discomfort. She gritted her teeth and flew past Tegla in the last few miles, en route to another first-place finish. That was as heroic an achievement as I've ever seen. When once asked why she runs the marathon, though, Uta simply answered, "I make the marathon beautiful for myself and for others. That's why I'm here."

I repeated that word, "beautiful," and looked out on the puzzled faces in my audience. Pain itself isn't beautiful, I said, but there is a beauty to effort, to perseverance, that marks it as special, as near as we may come to perfection.

I told them, too, of my own marathoning history. This is always a tricky business because I wanted to inspire them, not intimidate them. Many people find it easy to draw a distinction between what I've done and what they can do, saying that I must have some special gifts that enable me to accomplish these running feats. I told them that if I have any special gift, it's just stubbornness. There's nothing special about me that enables me to run so many races. My body might be a bit more durable than others, but there's really no reason why most of them couldn't run the same races that I do. All they need, I told them, is the determination to try. And despite my own experience, most people find that one marathon is plenty!

Some people nodded their heads, and some seem moved. Others sat politely in mute attention. Many of them joined our teams, and many did not. I always came away from these meetings with mixed emotions, feeling that I touched on something important, but that I'd circled rather than pierced the bulls-eye. I didn't manage to get to the heart of it; I couldn't fully explain what I felt. It was a frustrating, tiring business.

One moment crystallized my thinking. I had returned to Rome in 2002, and I had just finished pacing a group of my Team Diabetes runners to the finish line—marathon number 68 for me. Their day was over, but mine continued, as I ran back and forth on the course to cheer on the rest of my team and all the other race participants. I awaited two young women in particular: members of my team who were pushing against the clock. The race director, I knew, would shut off a section of the course at an appointed hour in order to let the city reclaim its streets, and the remaining runners on the course would have no choice but to cut the race short. It was a bum deal for those who had worked so hard and been struggling for so many hours, but there was no possibility for appeal. As I waited, I realized that my last two team members had not made the cutoff. They would cross the finish line, but they would not have completed 26.2 miles.

After the race, all of our teams from across the country returned to our host hotels, freshened up, and then gathered in the evening for a celebration dinner. There were smiles by the hundreds, and stories of obstacles overcome, random moments of hilarity, and new friendships forged. Above all, there was the electricity of accomplishment and pride. What-ever else may ever be said of them, they were now and forever marathoners.

But my two young women were not there. They were still upstairs in their shared room, and would not join us. Their marathon had been one of sacrifice and persistence without reward. They felt that they had nothing to celebrate. When I realized that they hadn't come down, I went up to talk with them.

I knocked on their door, and they let me in. I sat down, and asked how they were doing. Their words tumbled out in a flood, mixed with tears of frustration and anger. They spoke of their bitter disappointment, of the months of hard work they had poured into their dream, of their confidence in their ability to realize that dream if only it had *not been stolen from them*, of their dread of having to explain their failure to friends and family when they returned home. I sat and listened and tried to think of a way that I could tell them that there was nothing to be upset about, but I could not. It would be a lie.

But I did have something to say. I told them of the history of the race, of Phidippides's 25-mile journey, of the modern Olympic Games and the 1.2-mile accommodation to the British Royal family. I explained that the modern marathon is an exact distance, but that there is nothing sacred or immutable about the number 26.2. By itself it is without meaning; we alone give it meaning.

I spoke about time. I explained that my best time in a marathon is not the race in which I ranked highest; on that grand day in Detroit, I finished far behind the lead pack of runners, but I have never run faster. In other races, such as in Bermuda, I ran slower, but I finished higher in the final tally because my competitors were slower still. On which day, I asked them, was I the better runner? Of which day should I be proudest? I told them of my race in Pittsburgh, where I fought through heat and dehydration to finish over an hour slower I expected to. Rather than being despondent, though, I was thrilled with my performance that day, because I felt that I had shown courage.

So, I asked them, if distance doesn't matter, and time doesn't matter, what is the marathon about? What remains? In the end, what matters?

I spoke more about Detroit and Pittsburgh. Anyone can run well on a day when everything is in magical alignment, when your training has peaked, when injuries have been held at bay, when the course and the weather are perfect. Then performance is easy. In Detroit, I simply ran, like a machine. But in Pittsburgh, on the day when things were most difficult, when it would have been easiest to quit, that was the day when I asked more of myself than I thought I was able to give. It is in that kind of moment that glory can be found.

But in Rome, these two women had been denied their moment of glory. I told them that I knew that their victory had been stolen from them. But they had not given up. They had struggled, and had not turned away, even when they knew that they would ultimately not make the cutoff time, and would be rerouted on the course. There was no shame in what they had done, and their accomplishment was not lessened by the race director's decision. I told them that they had not completed a marathon; that was a simple fact that none of us could ignore. But they had not quit. They had transcended distance and time, and found something greater than just crossing a finish line; they had discovered the depth of their own power and determination. There would be other finish lines if they wanted them, as there were for me after my first disastrous marathon attempt, but they were already heroes, because they had journeyed and sacrificed and brought back the wisdom of self-knowledge.

We sat a while longer, and finally I stood up to leave. They thanked me earnestly, perhaps more for recognizing and validating their pain than for any other solace I tried to give them. As I walked away, I thought about what I had said, and tried to hold onto those thoughts the way you try to hold on to a dream upon waking. I felt that I had touched on something. This time, I had not become lost in a fog of words. This time, perhaps, I had moved just a step closer to finding the answer to my question.

In the meantime, I kept racing. Having tasted racing on foreign soil, it was all I really wanted to do. In March 2002, I raced Rome again, and then in April, I flew to Paris. I was certain that there was no better way to see a city than by running through it, and if there was one city that was big enough and beautiful enough to amaze runners over 26.2 miles, I was sure it would be Paris. But on race day, as I joined the 20,000 other runners gathered in the shadow of the Arc de Triomphe, I wondered whether it was fair of me to hold this race to such a high standard. It was a living city, not a museum showpiece, and this was a race, not a luxury tour. I tried to temper my expectations. There would be good parts and bad parts, I reminded myself, and all that I could be certain of was that eventually, if I kept moving forward, I would reach the finish line.

I needn't have worried. The City of Light turned out to be as glorious as I'd imagined it would be. After racing down the Champs-Élysées, we toured the parks and streets of the city, and then raced along the Seine. The Eiffel Tower loomed in the distance. It was breathtaking. Along the way I saw couples running in wedding attire, and heard shouts of *"Bon courage,"* and *"Allez! Allez!"* meaning, "Go! Go!" I later read in the *New York Times*[7] that spectators had taunted runners by shouting "Only 500 kilometers left!" and "Run faster! They're about to open the street up to cars!" According to the *Times*, the French appreciate track and field stars, but feel an ambivalence bordering on disdain for middle-of-the-pack runners. But I didn't hear any of those catcalls. Or maybe it was just that I don't speak French. For me, at least, marathon number 69 was perfect.

After returning from Paris, I settled into the morass of heat and humidity that is D.C. in the summertime. With temperatures climbing up into the 80s and 90s, there wasn't much for a marathoner to do; it was too hot for race organizers to safely hold any long distance events in all but the most northern of cities, or in chilly San Francisco, which is no surprise to anyone who's been there in July. So summer usually stretches out into a long season of training and catching up with running friends. And of making plans for the smorgasbord of fall races.

My grandmother used to have a saying: you make plans and God laughs. She was about to be proven right.

---

7 April 14, 2002, p.10.

Running and Romance

I have to admit it: my love for running marathons required a certain amount of understanding from the women I dated. We marathoners are a tough group for nonrunners to understand. We train our bodies for our own health and vanity, and then race to prove to ourselves how tough we are. Every day's activities are planned around the run. Friends and families sometimes take a back seat. Like most marathoners, I didn't really see anything wrong with this. I thought it was fair for me to have a space in my life that was all my own. As long as I didn't ignore any responsibilities, I didn't see anything wrong with doing what I wanted to do.

Unless, of course, I wanted to share my life with someone else. Most women who at first were attracted to my passion for running soon tired of my priorities. My getting up at 5 A.M. to run or meet with personal training clients, and fading by 9 or 10 at night, didn't help either. Eventually, they all asked why I couldn't just sit down and relax.

On occasion I dated another runner. It seemed like the natural thing to do: find someone who shared my passion and interest. All of my friends expected this of me; what could be more natural than for a marathoner to be involved with another marathoner?

As it turned out, it wasn't really that simple. Learning to date and train with someone as active as myself raised new issues. We all define ourselves in many different ways. For me, being a marathon runner is a big part of who I am. The athletic women I dated felt the same way, but sometimes their emotional lives were more complex. One woman in particular that I dated had always been the athletic alpha partner, faster and fitter than her dates. In this important arena, success defined her as a person. Things were different when I came along. Suddenly, she wasn't the one who could run or bike farther and faster, and she wasn't used to that. Whether we realized it or not, we weren't just romantically involved, we were competitors. Even as she tried to hide it, resentment and anger grew, and spilled out in small ways, and I didn't know how to handle it. After all, *I* didn't feel the need to compete with *her*. But it was easy for me to feel this way, since I wasn't the one having my self-image challenged. Would I feel comfortable if she was a better runner than I was? I'd like to think so, but I don't know for sure.

Ultimately, that relationship didn't work out, and not just for that reason, but it did play a part. I knew that things didn't have to be like that in every dual-athlete relationship; there were plenty of successful running couples out there. It just wasn't happening for me. But that was okay. I didn't feel the urgent need to settle down anyway.

But I did want a special person in my life someday, and to have a home and family: the whole nine yards. Suddenly, that person entered my life. Or rather, re-entered. It was Stephanie Kay, the former high school classmate from Boston whom I had tried to contact years before. Our class was now about to mark its twentieth graduation anniversary. Some class members had set up a Web site, and e-mails were flying in all directions. I thought I'd give it one more shot, so I sent her an e-mail. She wrote back. I answered, and then so did she. She told me that she had gotten my message years earlier, and had wanted to call me back, but that my message had been lost at her office. We now exchanged phone numbers, and had hours-long conversations about running and art and anything we could think of. One night, as we spoke on the phone, we hit a natural stopping point. There was just nothing else that came to mind to say. I expected her to wrap things up, but instead she waited on the phone for wherever our conversation would go next. It hit me right then: she liked me.

It was a long time coming, actually. I first met her back in 1976, when we both entered junior high school together in New York City. I was just twelve, and was immediately smitten, but at that tender age I was too shy and inexperienced to know what to do about it. So I did nothing.

The years passed, and although I never managed to ask Stephanie out, I did manage to become friends with her. Finally, we were in twelfth grade—seniors at last! Our senior trip was a ski weekend, and one night, as several of us were relaxing after a long day of skiing, I managed to finally ask her for a date. Sort of. I asked if she'd like to take a walk in the woods with me. With hindsight I can see how this could have seemed a little too bold. Stephanie must have thought so, because she politely declined. Later, she wrote some nice things in my yearbook, but signed it "wuv." Sadly, the replacement of that "L" with a "W" told me all that I needed to know about her feelings for me.

And now, all these years later, we were talking, and then making plans to meet up in New York. Then she visited me in D.C., and I visited her in Boston. By the time the reunion came around we were a couple. Little by little her "W" turned into an "L."

I had come to think of D.C. as my home, but the more time I spent with Stephanie in Boston, the more I grew to love it there. Which is not to say that every visit was like a fairy tale come true. For example, that summer I went up to visit her for the July 4th weekend. We avoided the throngs of people mobbed along the Charles River to watch the fireworks and hear the Boston Pops, but the next morning was clear and beautiful; a perfect day for an easy 8-mile run along the river. Evidence of the previous evening's celebration was everywhere, although cleanup crews were already hard at work emptying overstuffed trash cans and picking up litter, oblivious to the runners and cyclists flying past them.

Along the bicycle trail sat row upon row of portable toilets, put in place over the previous several days to handle the crush of revelers. Now, like cannons left on a battlefield, they sat silent, but apparently still usable. I don't usually have access to such conveniences except on race day; my training runs are often marked by moments of brilliant improvisation in dealing with bathroom issues. But now, faced with such opulence, I decided to use one of the silent soldiers.

I swung open the door on the nearest Porta-Jon. Just as I was getting comfortable, I heard the sound of a truck nearby. Very nearby. Suddenly I felt the stall move. I jumped to my feet and grabbed at the door, but it was pinned shut by the long metal arms of the truck's hydraulic lift. I was trapped!

I wasn't sure whether to laugh or scream. I opted for shouting, and after several tense moments of yelling and peering out of the mesh screen at the top of the stall, I finally caught the driver's attention. He motioned to me to stay put—where would I possibly go?—and he moved the truck so that I could free myself from my little prison. As I resumed my run under the bemused gaze of the driver, I wondered whether anyone would believe what had just happened to me. What if I couldn't get the driver's attention? Is there a secret Porta-John burial ground? Would it be more than a days' run from where I was staying in Boston? Would Stephanie recognize me if I even made it back to her? Would she want to?

But luckily, I made it back to Stephanie safe and sound, and we continued our courtship.

And that's how I found myself one afternoon at the top of Old Rag Mountain in the Shenandoahs, about to get down on one knee. It was a beautiful, sunny day, with a nice crispness in the air. I had packed a lunch, including chocolates with strawberries, and a bottle of wine. And a diamond ring. My plan was to find just the right spot; someplace sheltered from the wind, but bathed in sunshine, with a sweeping view of the valley below. And I found it. Everything was perfect. I began to set out our lunch.

Just then a young woman and a few men passed by. We exchanged hellos, and then I heard a loud thud. The woman had fallen heavily while jumping from one rock to another, and had twisted her ankle badly. Right next to our spot. I suddenly had a vision of all my carefully laid plans going up in smoke. I reached into my bag for an ace bandage.

"Would you like to wrap your ankle, so you can *get going*?"

"No," she said. "But it hurts so much, I'm feeling nauseous."

Nauseous. Right next to our perfect spot. I waited twenty years for this moment, and now this woman is going to throw up on us.

"Would you like some water, so you can *get going*?"

"Ugh," she said. "I'm seeing spots."

Spots. I couldn't believe it.

"That must be the altitude," I told her. Look, I know the Shenandoahs are not the Himalayas, but I was improvising. "You need to be at a lower altitude. You really should *get going*."

Finally, I realized that this woman wasn't going to be able to move anytime soon. Her friends were helping her, so I wasn't needed, but I would have to change my plan. Luckily, Stephanie and I were able to find another suitable spot, and this time there were no interruptions when, all these years after I had asked her to walk in the woods with me, I asked her my second bold question.

And this time she said "yes."

Running Tip #13

Strength Training

There are runners who believe fervently in strength training, while others argue just as strongly against it. I'm a believer; strength training helps maintain good bone density, and running efficiency, and keeps injuries at a minimum.

- *Invest in some expert advice.* Paying a personal trainer to show you the right way to do your exercises is money well spent.
- *Always change your routine.* This keeps you and your body from getting bored, and provides the best stimulus to your body for adaptation, so alternate between free weights, cables, machines, and body-weight movements.
- *Work the core.* Any exercise that forces you to balance will work muscles crucial to your running, including your abdominals, lower back, glutes, and hip stabilizers.
- *Do complex movements.* The more joints you get involved, the more muscles you'll be training. So forget bicep curls; do some squats and push-ups.
- *Don't rest; alternate body parts.* You've got the endurance for this, so use it, and get your workout over in lightning speed.

A Race Like No Other

My fall 2002 racing campaign began with a solid run in the Toronto Marathon in September, followed by the Portland Marathon in early October, which enabled me to add Oregon to my list of states completed. Portland's race was as scenic and well-organized as any of the other dozens of marathons I'd run, but what stood out in my mind was a short, brutal climb up and over a short suspension bridge, and the tiny redwood saplings the volunteers handed out to finishers at the end of the race. The rest of the country had not yet added "carbon footprint" to their lingo, but Portland was way ahead of them.

Two weeks after crossing the finish line in Portland, I flew out to Amsterdam with a small team of Arthritis Foundation charity fundraisers. Little by little, I was working my way to Europe's greatest cities, and each one was proving to be more astonishing than the last. I loved Amsterdam for its streets and canals and museums, and yes, even its redlight district and marijuana-selling coffee shops, though I was too shy and conservative to do more than quickly walk past either. More to my liking was the wonderful Van Gogh Museum. There was also the famous Rijksmuseum to stroll through, as well as a somber visit to the house of

Anne Frank, the young victim of the Holocaust whose memoirs touched the world.

But I had other things on my mind as well. I was especially looking forward to the race; Amsterdam's marathon course had once held the marathon world record, and was reputed to be as beautiful as it was flat and fast. But the day before the marathon I fell ill with a bad cold, and on race day I felt miserable. Still, after traveling all that way to be with my team and run the race, I wasn't about to let a cold stop me.

The cold had other ideas. By the halfway point, I knew that I wouldn't be able to run the entire race, and that I'd be lucky to even finish as a walker. Still, I pressed on, running as much as I could, and walking the rest. As I stumbled on, I tried to appreciate the beauty of the course. It had meandered through the downtown area, then wandered to the outskirts of town, passing along a river and old windmills. It's often difficult to be objective about a racecourse when you've had a rough day; it's too tempting to think badly of a race in which you performed badly. But in Amsterdam, it was easy to see that despite my own difficulties, it was a wonderful race. I only regretted that I wasn't able to make the most of it.

Even in my depleted condition, however, I found myself trying to push as hard as I could. Seeing other walkers brought out my competitive juices, and I silently took aim at each one directly in front of me, quickening my pace to catch and pass them. It might sound compulsive, but this helped me feel like I was still part of a race, even as my expected finishing time soared higher than I ever thought it could be. When at long last I crossed the finish line, though, I wasn't concerned about my time; I was just thrilled that I had managed to go on when it would have been so easy to quit. It was a lesson I had learned before, but which was worth learning again: some of my best moments aren't my fastest moments.

Marathon number 72 was in the books.

Two weeks after running Amsterdam, I ran the New York City Marathon again. I had beaten my cold, and was ready for a real race.

But even with all I had experienced in fifteen years of racing, there were still some things to learn. For example, I had believed it to be impossible to urinate while running. To the extent that I had ever thought about it—and I know that by thinking about it at all I am among 1/100th of 1 percent of people on the planet—I had thought it was like keeping your eyes open while sneezing: theoretically possible, but not likely to be seen in my lifetime.

As it turned out, I was wrong. The race had just started, and all of us in our tens of thousands were huffing our way up the Verrazano Bridge, when I noticed some runners to my right who were transfixed with something just ahead of us. They seemed amazed. I saw why: a woman wearing nylon shorts was letting go as she ran. Besides being inconsiderate of those of us behind her—and was there ever a better incentive to pick up the pace and pass someone?—I couldn't imagine running 25 more miles on a crisp November morning in those soaked shorts. But maybe she had once had a bad Porta-Jon experience, too.

But that wasn't my problem. In fact I had few problems at all that day, and I was rewarded with a finishing time almost an hour faster than I had just posted in the Netherlands.

And then two weeks after that, I ran a local race in Maryland. It was a cold, wet day, and when I crossed the finish line, I was relieved to see that the race organizers had put out soup and pizza to revive us. I was famished, and stacked three slices of pizza one atop the other, downing them all at once like a big hoagie. I'm glad the race photographers didn't capture that moment.

Two weeks after *that* race, I returned to Hawaii with another charity team to run the Honolulu Marathon. On the flight home, I thought about how, after fifteen years of marathoning, my body seemed to need less and less recovery time. I didn't know exactly how this had happened, but my body had obviously adapted on a very fundamental level.

The marathons kept coming. Number 76: Miami; number 77: Boston, number 78: Kona, Hawaii.

Ah, Kona. A race obviously dreamed up by a sadist who knew nothing about running. It was held on the Big Island of Hawaii, which sounds like a tropical paradise to anyone who hasn't been there. To those in the know, however, most of the island is a hot, barren lava field. A friend of mine had run it the year before and had lost eight of her toenails due to swelling of her feet during the race. I had already weathered plenty of hot-weather racing, so I knew what to expect and how to handle it, but for the uninitiated—that is, for the virgin marathoners on my charity team—it was a brutal awakening. I tired to help them understand what they were up against, but no amount of talking was going to fully prepare them for the broiling moonscape on which they found themselves. I stayed on the course helping our runners—and anyone else I saw in difficulty—until our very last participant crossed the finish line. As much as I love the marathon, I think the best that could be said of this one is that we all managed to get through it.

After Kona, I believed that I had pretty much figured out the marathon. The scenery might change from race to race, the temperatures and elevation might vary, and the crowds might differ in size and enthusiasm, but the overall experience would usually be the same. There would be an adrenaline rush at the blast of the starting gun. There would be early optimism, shouts of support, and periodic aid stations. There would be eventual fatigue, and perhaps blisters. There would inevitably be a moment of truth, accompanied by a wave of determination, and then perseverance, culminating with euphoria at the finish line. This is the beauty of the marathon—its predictability, and its simplicity. You just run 26.2 miles as fast as you can, and if you do it right, there are usually precious few shocks along the way.

Or so I thought. Then I read about a marathon that is different from all the others, the name of which brings a smile to the face of those who are in the know: the Marathon des Châteaux du Médoc, or as it is more commonly and simply called, Médoc. If the marathon is the serious-minded older sibling of running, then Médoc is the wild child, looking for the nearest party. In a sport defined by discipline, Médoc is the Dionysian exception: a race that is more revelry than competition.

Created in 1985 as a tour for a group of athletic wine connoisseurs, the race is a September jaunt along roads and trails, past fifty-nine vineyards in Pauillac, in the Bordeaux region of southern France, by the shores of the river Gironde. To say that it is just a race through wine country, though, is like saying that Mardi Gras is just a celebration of Fat Tuesday, because the organizers have turned the marathon into a uniquely local creation; a celebration of the senses. It has become famous for wine, food and music stations along the course, and for the outlandish costumes worn by its participants. Even the race materials caution you to think of it as more of a tour than a competition. It is truly what Ernest Hemingway named Paris: a moveable feast.

I first learned about Médoc in the mid-90s in a newspaper article that took a "look what those crazy foreigners are up to now" approach to reporting on the race. The race was described as being more notable for the quantities of wine and oysters consumed than for fast times produced. While most marathons are a 26-mile adventure, Médoc sounded more like it needed a twelve-step program, but I was more intrigued than dismayed. I knew that some day I would have to experience it for myself.

Several obstacles became immediately apparent, starting with simply getting into the race. Like most chronic marathoners, I had become accustomed to having to compete with other applicants to get a number in the most popular races. Over the years, the Marine Corps Marathon began to fill up more and more quickly, and soon would close out within days of being open, while New York required split second timing just to get a race application considered. Still, these races offered enough slots to give most runners hope: 18,000, 25,000, or 35,000. Not so with Médoc. The narrow lanes along which the course meanders makes a huge field of marathoners impossible, so the race is limited to only 8,000 participants. It is also an immensely popular race, and registration closes out quickly. To race Médoc, you have to commit early and keep your fingers crossed.

In April 2002, when I traveled to Paris, I thought I had managed a particularly good coup at the marathon expo: I convinced a race official at the Médoc Marathon information booth to let me reserve a block of one dozen slots for my running friends and myself. I thought it would be an easy sell back home. The race official put his initials on an application and told me to send it in with payment for the reserved slots as soon as possible. I was so pleased with my good fortune that I sent in the money while I was still in France. But when I got back to the States, a voice mail message was waiting for me that said, in a thick French accent, that there was a problem with my race application. Not trusting phone contact, I sent an e-mail explaining the arrangement I had worked out with the race official. All settled, I thought. Then I received an e-mail in return telling me that my demand to talk to the race director was refused. I was confused. Obviously, this was going to be more complicated than I thought, especially since I didn't speak French.

As I tried to sort out the application process, I also began to consider the logistics. There weren't any direct flights from the United States to Bordeaux. The best that I could arrange was to fly direct to Paris, and then either take a connecting flight or a bullet train to Bordeaux. And on arrival, the difficulties don't end; Pauillac is far from the Bordeaux city center, and lodging there is very limited. The only workable option seemed to be to stay in the city and arrange for a driver to take me for the nearly hour and a half long ride to the race start.

Ultimately, my plans to run Médoc collapsed that year like a house of cards. Still, I had caught the scent, and I would not give up hope. And then suddenly, in 2003, the opportunity arose: Jenice Cunningham, a coach and team coordinator for the Arthritis Foundation based in Atlanta, was putting together a team. I knew Jenice from the Honolulu, Dublin, and Amsterdam marathons. Jenice had worked out all the details, and she had called me to find out if I wanted to come along. I answered yes before she was even finished asking the question.

With the logistics all taken care of, I settled into deciding on a training plan. Knowing that Médoc is no ordinary marathon, I wondered if I needed to alter my usual routine. Speed work is usually a part of my regular marathon preparation, and speed can pay off handsomely in Médoc, where I had heard rumors that the winner in each age category receives his or her weight in wine. I'm not an elite runner, though, so a fast marathon would leave me without the winner's prize and also without full enjoyment of the race's amenities. Even if I could somehow miraculously take first place, I didn't think I would be able to survive the reward, even with the help of my friends. I decided on a more leisurely approach to the race. I crossed speed work off my to-do list. So far, so good.

The next issue was thornier. How does one prepare to drink wine during a race? I considered adding alcohol to my training regimen, but I was unable to find any advice on how to do this. Should I slowly increase my intake week to week, along with my mileage? Would it matter what kind of wine I trained with? I scrapped the whole idea; I just would build up a solid running base and let the race-day drinking take care of itself.

Although I couldn't find any information on training for Médoc, I did find plenty of advice on how to actually run the race. The first suggestion I came across was to skip wine altogether for the first half of the race, on the theory that if I should then encounter any ill effects from wine tasting, I would be close enough to the end to successfully make it across the finish line. The second tip was to not actually swallow the wine. Instead, I was told to just swirl the wine in my mouth like a professional taster, and then spit it out. This would theoretically give me the pleasure of experiencing the wine without actually getting drunk, the reasoning being, I presume, that being drunk diminishes the chances of crossing the finish line. A third idea was to simply run the race in a straightforward, no-funny-business manner—no wine, no food, no partying. Then, after coming across the finish line, I could make my way back on to the course to eat and drink to my heart's content.

These all seemed like very well-reasoned strategies. Naturally, I ignored them all. I had decided against running Médoc carefully and strategically; that just didn't seem to be true to the spirit of the race. Spitting out wine must be a kind of heresy in France, and as for backtracking the course, when my legs cross a finish line, they know the race is over, and they don't like to run after that. I decided to experience the race fully and let the chips fall where they may.

There was, however, one more issue I would have to consider before making my way to the starting line: what to wear. Usually this is a simple matter: shorts and singlet in warm weather, graduating through different combinations until I came to tights, gloves and a hat, with a long-sleeved top and jacket, in the coldest weather. Médoc, of course, demanded a different approach. The race materials not only mentioned that most participants wear a costume, but also promised an extra prize for all participants who did so.

What's that old phrase? In for a penny, in for a pound. Everyone in my group—myself included—decided that we would go the extra mile, so to speak, and wear a costume. But whatever we chose would have to be not only eye-catching, but practical as well. After all, this wasn't just some Halloween bash or a Thanksgiving Turkey Trot; we would have to wear this costume for 26.2 miles. With that in mind, Jenice's group agreed on the perfect outfit: grass skirts and leis over our running duds. I daringly cut the skirt down to make it more suitable for running—almost a grass miniskirt, really. I smiled at the incongruity of seeing it lying next to my usual race gear, but I began to relax. All the big issues were now decided.

Finally, September rolled around, and I found myself boarding a jet for a red-eye flight to Paris. I arrived almost too tired to appreciate the gleaming glass and steel of Charles de Gaulle airport as I made my way to my connecting flight. In the months since I committed to the race, international events had stormed onto the front pages as we moved closer toward war with Iraq. I wondered whether the rift between the U.S. and French governments would affect my travel and race plans, and whether Americans would no longer find themselves welcome in Bordeaux. I've long believed in the spiritual healing power of a marathon, but this was a tall order. Could wine, food, and running bring us together? I'd soon find out.

My flight landed in Bordeaux without incident, and if I had any doubts about where I was, they were quickly dispelled as giant bottles of cabernet sauvignon stared down at us from atop the baggage carousels. After a short ride to our hotel and a quick check-in, several of us went out for a walkabout.

Bordeaux seemed to be in the early stages of a renaissance, with ongoing restoration and construction projects throughout the city center. Its old-world charm was still evident, though, as cafes, restaurants, and shops lined the streets in centuries-old stone buildings, all leading down to the wide Gironde River. The streets looked impossibly narrow, and the traffic was choking, but to us, it was a beautiful place. We were even able to find a place that served pizza—or, at least, a version of it. And better still, we located a nearby supermarket for loading up on water and fresh fruit.

The following morning we piled into our chartered bus for the hour-long drive out to Pauillac for the race expo and number pickup. After entering the athletic center that served as race headquarters, we encountered a small sample of what to expect the next day, as an older gentleman in full American Indian costume stared us down at the entryway, and made folks jump by periodically letting out a short war whoop. Being a city boy, I admit to only a sketchy knowledge of Native Americans, but even I knew this was very odd. It would prove to be only the first of many such moments.

We proceeded to get our numbers, shirts, and race timing chips. Having a chip in a race like this seemed out of place; it was one of the few telltale signs that this was an actual competition at all. We then made our way to the modest Médoc Marathon expo. A few other races, including the Chicago Marathon, were represented, and among the race memorabilia that was available for purchase were bottles of wine with the race logo emblazoned on the label. There was also another uniquely Médoc concession tucked in among the stalls: a costume seller catering to those who hadn't yet settled on a race day outfit. As I looked over the racks of Viking, maiden, and clown costumes, I realized that my team's Hawaiian ensemble would probably seem very conservative compared to what we would see the next day.

I mulled that over as we went back to Bordeaux and spent the day lounging around waiting for our pasta feed. The race organizers put on their own prerace dinner—complete with copious amount of *le vin*, of course—but we opted to be closer to our hotel and an early bedtime. Though the race was scheduled to start at 9:30 A.M., the long drive necessary to get there required a predawn departure. Far from being annoyed, I was almost soothed by this return to a slice of my usual prerace regimen.

The next morning I scarfed down a light, high-carb breakfast, then boarded the bus and settled into a doze as the sun rose over the French countryside. The air was crisp and just a bit cool, with temperatures nudging into the 60s.

Stepping out of the bus in Pauillac, I couldn't help but think of the colorful world into which Dorothy's house fell in *The Wizard of Oz*. All around me were odd characters in running shoes; mimes, devils, cavemen, bunnies, pirates, prisoners sporting a helium ball and chain, cats and mice, and all manner of cartoon characters. There was face paint galore, and even teams of runners pulling theme carts, like mini floats in a Thanksgiving Day parade.

I had read that 70 percent of the participants were costumed, but on race day it felt like a much higher percentage; it seemed not just like many people had a costume, but rather that virtually everyone had one. Dressing in a plain running outfit suddenly seemed like a mortal sin, and I was glad that my team had at least made an effort, humble as it was. As I walked past a row of portable toilets, though, I wondered how all these odd and otherworldly people would manage the details and necessities of running a race. No matter; we were a colorful group, and we were having a good time.

In fact, we were the most self-aware race group I'd ever seen. In the minutes before most races, runners seem lost in their own thoughts, full of nervous energy about the challenge they would soon face. In Médoc, though, the prerace mood was festive; it was all about people-watching, preening, and enjoying yourself. There were dancers gyrating on platforms above the crowd, and everybody was posing and snapping photos of those around them. A Japanese group, dressed as samurai, even had their own camera crew following them around the starting line to record their encounters with other outlandish runners. It all reminded me of the crowd I'd seen at Grateful Dead shows years ago, which was so happy to just be there that watching the band almost seemed like an afterthought. Watching us laugh and point at one another at the starting line, it was almost easy to forget that we would soon be running a marathon.

But there was indeed a race, and suddenly we were off. We wound our way out of town, past scenic storefronts and booths offering food and wine-tasting, and past cheering supporters. We made our way toward the vineyards, and soon came upon the first official aid stop, just a few kilometers into the race. It was amply supplied with water, cake, cookies, raisins, dried apricots, and even prunes—prunes, for heaven's sake!—but no wine. In fact, there was no wine at any of the early aid stops. I wondered whether the race directors thought it best to protect us from ourselves. As the sun poked its way though and the temperature began to climb, I began to think this might not have been a bad decision.

Kilometer 9 brought our first wine-tasting opportunity. I was treated to the unusual sight of tables lined up with glass after glass of dark red Bordeaux. Never has being a runner seemed so rewarding! I slowed to a walk and lifted a glass. As I savored the first sip, I knew that I wouldn't remember the taste of the wine or even the vineyard, but I'd certainly remember the sensation. I tossed the glass in a receptacle and resumed running.

As we made or way past the châteaux and back into the fields, I saw a number of runners split from the pack and head out between the rows of grapes. It took me a moment to realize that they were taking bathroom breaks. A runner would not be surprised at such behavior, but I bet that wine connoisseurs would certainly be shocked.

We continued through the French countryside, passing the occasional stone châteaux and cyclists on holiday. We ran on paved roads, but more frequently on dirt paths alongside the vines, the pounding of our feet kicking up the soft, powdery dirt into low clouds. We didn't come across another wine-tasting stop until kilometer 16, but there were plenty of aid stations along the way offering refreshments and cool, wet sponges. The sun was shining brightly by this time, and I was starting to wonder about how the heat would affect our ragtag group. As if on command, some dark clouds rolled in, bringing along a welcome sprinkle of drizzle that cooled us off and quieted the billowing dust around our feet. The drizzle continued, however, and grew in strength, and soon became rain. Usually a cause for disgruntlement, the rain instead became a cause for more drinking.

At some point along this part of the marathon I had the most unusual sensation; I thought I saw flowers blowing around me, as if a herald were scattering petals in my path. Perhaps I was having a bad reaction to the wine. But no. Slowly recognition creased my bewildered brain—my lei had broken, and was quickly dispersing itself. I gathered up the loose ends and tied them together tightly. Just as my grass skirt had been short-ened, my lei was now a streamlined version of its former self.

We also began to come across bands along the course offering up some musical distractions. Oddly enough, when I passed a couple of them, they were playing old American country and rockabilly tunes, like "Blue Moon of Kentucky." Not exactly what you'd expect to hear a band playing in France, but sometimes it's better to just appreciate a moment than to ask why and how.

After the second wine stop, the tastings came more frequently, and I stuck with my promise to taste each and every wine that they put in our path. Soon I lost count, but I knew that in all, there would be twenty-one wine-tasting stations. I've never been a math whiz, but even I could fig-ure out that with there being only two wine stops in the first half of the race, there would be quite a bit of catching up to do. I mustered my best bit of marathoner's determination for the task that lay ahead.

As I continued on my way, I also realized something else about the course: its sheer beauty. I knew that it wasn't just the alcohol talking as I wondered whether this might not be the most beautiful marathon course I've ever run. It wasn't just that there were breathtaking sights along the way, although there were plenty of those. It was the absence of something; the inevitable marathon dead zone, the dry spot to be found in all races, where we labor though industrial parks, past train tracks and factories and parking lots, with no supporters to cheer us on, and no eye candy to distract us from our boredom and suffering. Boston has such a zone, lined by railroad tracks. So does the New York Marathon, in Queens, before hitting the Queensboro Bridge. And so do countless other races. But in Médoc, I realized, there was nothing but row after row of grapevines, full with their dark fruit, and beautiful châteaux lording over their fields.

The beauty of the course and the glory of the wine couldn't stave off the realities of running a marathon, however, and despite my leisurely early pace, I began to slow in the second part of the race. I won't blame it all on the wine, not when there were also some other obstacles I could point my finger at, like the food. At one station I took a bit of unidentified food and shoved it into my mouth. After all, no one would put out food on a marathon course that would be bad for us, right? Wrong, I realized too late. Wrong, wrong, wrong. Of all the foods in the world, the only one that I truly hate was liver. What I had now in my mouth was some type of liver-based lunchmeat. Yuck. The memory of it still haunts me, and has led me to instituting a new racing rule: put nothing in your mouth that you can't identify. My mother later insisted that she taught me that rule years ago, though I'm not so sure about that.

The race continued onward, past kilometers 25, 30, and 35. Then, at kilometer number 38, with just four kilometers to go, the race let loose, like a child that's been quiet too long and needs to scream. First came the oysters, piled ostentatiously on serving tables. A teammate of mine later told me of a writer's observation: "Oh, the courage of the first brave soul to slurp an oyster!" On that day in Bordeaux, I can tell you, there were plenty of brave men and women, and I struggled to be among the bravest.

Next up was a steak station, where bits of grilled beef on sticks were served up to runners. I took just a small piece to taste, then moved on to the next station just down the road, the cheese tables! And after that, more wine! I gulped and chewed and gulped some more, and then, as I slowly fell back into an easy running pace, a little voice somewhere deep inside began telling me that my gluttony wasn't such a great idea. I slowed down a little more as the oysters began to talk to me, and I reminded myself that I only had a little over 1 kilometer to go. I also said a little prayer of thanks to the race directors for not putting the oysters in the first half of the race.

One last unexpected race amenity awaited runners who made it this far: face paint. For those who had been too shy to wear a costume, or who had somehow lost it along the way, there was a chance for last-minute redemption. A couple of volunteers were quickly dabbing color onto runners on request. I opted for some black and red stripes down my nose and across my cheeks. All I can say is that it seemed like a good idea at the time.

And finally, the finish line was just up ahead. As I crossed through, I was given a backpack with the race logo on it, and a bottle of wine to put in it. For my costume-wearing efforts, I was also given a fanny pack bearing the race logo. And last but not least, I was pointed toward the finisher's tent, where wine and beer were being freely doled out. Perhaps not surprisingly, I had had enough by this point, and as appreciative as I was of the postrace offerings, I decided to head to the bus instead. And probably not in a straight line, either, despite my best efforts.

The afternoon was spent recovering from the race, followed later by more wine and food. The next day, we all decided to partake of the vineyard walk offered to race participants, featuring—you guessed it— more wine and food. A highlight was the lunch tent set up at the end of the tour, where oysters and other fare were doled out as a French chanteuse belted out old American tunes and various national anthems. Somehow, I wasn't at all surprised. By this time, I had learned to expect the unexpected.

After the race, we took a train back to Paris—still drinking along the way, of course. We then spent a few days drying out and sightseeing. As I gazed at the now-familiar Eiffel Tower and wandered the Latin Quarter, I tried to put the race in perspective. It seemed to fit into no readily available category. It belonged in a category all its own.

The winners of the marathon, incidentally, posted times of 2:32:52 for the men and 2:56:27 for the women; entirely respectable finishing times that seemed incongruous with my own experience. My finishing time was just about the slowest I've ever had—let's just say it was between four and five hours. Still, it was good enough to put me first in my little group; this was probably more of a reflection of the party instinct of my group than my own speed. But my slow time seemed to show the truth behind the race's motto: below an image of an apparently snookered runner weaving from pillar to post is the phrase "Médoc, Le Marathon Le Plus Long Du Monde," "Médoc, the Longest Marathon in the World." While it might have felt like an ultramarathon, I knew that Médoc is not really a race to be measured in time, or perhaps even by distance. It really was like no other race in the world.

As much fun as racing in Bordeaux proved to be, it wasn't the only excitement I had running that September. There was Hurricane Isabel to consider. It started as a small updraft as water evaporated over warm south Atlantic waters. The updraft gathered strength and grew into a tropical storm, and then flexed its muscles and grew into a Category 5 hurricane, with winds raging at 160 miles per hour. Inexorably, it moved toward the Carolina coast, and up toward Washington, D.C. Naturally, I took that as a sign to lace up my training shoes for the run of a lifetime.

As the storm drew near, batteries and bottled water were cleaned off store shelves, and schools, as well as federal and local government agencies, announced that they would be closed. Thursday—hurricane day—started out gray and windy, and I felt a sense of expectation among those out on the streets, rushing through last-minute preparations. As the day ebbed into evening, the winds picked up to a howl, and rain swept through in waves. The storm was drawing near, and it was almost time for me to go.

It was 9:30 p.m. when I finally ventured outside. The first thing I noticed was how very warm it was. It must have been in the upper

80s, and I immediately regretted bringing a light jacket. The rain had let up, and the winds had died down a bit as I ran southwest toward the Potomac River. If there were a front-row seat to the storm, it would be on one of the city's bridges, where wind can whip over the open water like race cars at Daytona.

As I ran down the city streets, I passed shuttered and boarded businesses, but also some open bars and restaurants, catering to the adventurous, the bored, or the addicted. There were already a few trees down, and debris littered the road. A handful of taxis roamed the streets, and there were a few police cruisers out, but little else. I ran down the center of M Street in the Georgetown district, one of the busiest thoroughfares in the city, and I was all alone. It was the first time I'd ever been able to do that. I felt giddy with power; this storm was not as bad as I thought it would be. Clearly, Isabel had lost a great deal of her punch as she made her way inland. Just then, a branch swatted me across the back of my head, as if to remind me that the storm had not yet lost all of its teeth.

I turned onto Key Bridge and looked across the Potomac River toward Virginia. I was about a third of the way across when the big winds hit. I was blown from side to side of the walkway like a pinball, despite my best efforts to run a straight line. As wind whipped my face, I found it difficult to breathe. It was exhilarating, but also terrifying, and it occurred that it wouldn't take very much more wind to send me hurtling over the railing for a hundred-foot plunge into the river below. I made it to the other side, then turned to head back home. My ambitious 12-mile course had been cut to a short 5-miler, but that was enough of a taste of the hurricane for me.

As I neared my apartment, the storm picked up in intensity, as if to say that it had only been toying with me so far, and that it was now ready to really play. Rain began to pour down again, and the wind increased. I raced toward my building and burst through the doors like it was the tape in a 5K race, then stood there, dripping and panting as the storm raged on the other side of the glass door like a lion in a cage. By that time, Stephanie had moved down to D.C. and was living with me. She just handed me a towel and shook her head.

By morning, the storm was all but spent. I ran different trails during the following days to assess the damage. Fallen trees across one of my favorite bike paths made for a unique climbing-running duathlon. Friends in the suburbs reported that their power was out, and would be for at least another week, from what they'd been told. Still, the city had been lucky to escape with relatively little damage; it has been far luckier than many other coastal towns. And I was lucky to have unwittingly found a relatively gentle hour during the storm to squeeze in my hurricane run.

Running Tip #14

The Bathroom Break

One thing that sets runners apart is the utilitarian view we take of our bodies. We see them as machines, built through training for high performance. Our need to relieve ourselves before a race is usually no more embarrassing to us than a need to check the oil in our car. This might put us at odds with the rest of the civilized world, but we're okay with that. Still, there are basic guidelines to follow to avoid any problems in this area.

- *Deal with bodily needs before the race begins.* All major marathons provide hundreds of Porta-Jons at their race starts, but before a race, the lines to get in one are usually very long. Minimize your need for them by cutting off the fluid intake a full hour before the race start. Wait until just 5 minutes before the race is to begin, then gulp down 6–8 ounces of water or sports drink.

- *Don't be too shy during the race.* Marathoners tend to act with unspoken cooperation during a race; we keep an eye out for places other runners choose to use. But sometimes, a race course simply doesn't provide any secluded spots to take care of business. Like Superman without a phone booth, I've sometimes found myself looking in horror at fields without trees and city streets without dark alleys, and those are somehow also the spots where the crowds of spectators seems most dense. In such situations, do what you must. Remember: during a marathon, the regular rules of proper public behavior don't apply.

→

Running Tip #14

If you doubt me, think of marathon world record–holder Paula Radcliffe, who, en route to winning the London Marathon in April 2004, crouched down on the course to relieve herself. She apologized afterward, but runners knew no apology was necessary. We understood.

A Bit of Hardware

By 2004, I had run eighty-four marathons, and my collection of medals was something to see. My first medal was earned in the Marine Corps Marathon in 1987, and though I was fiercely proud of it at the time, I can now admit that it was a cheap little thing. It was fashioned to resemble a dog tag, but looked like it had been pulled from a cereal box. As the race matured over the years, though, and received corporate sponsorship, its medals improved, and now they're smart, gleaming works of running art.

Twelve years later, when I crossed the finish line in Antarctica, I didn't get a finisher's medal at all. I wasn't concerned, though, because all of the runners were told that medals would be mailed to our homes later. Sure enough, it showed up in my mailbox a few weeks after I'd returned home. It was the biggest, heaviest, and gaudiest medal I had ever seen. I was thrilled; it was a tangible reminder of where I had been and what I had accomplished. But receiving a medal was not a surprise; most marathoners—even many elite runners—work so hard with so little tangible reward that we have come to expect, even demand, that we be given a finisher's medal upon completing the course. And in commenting on a race, a description of the medal is often right up there with reviews of the course and the race support. And woe to the race director who fails to deliver; he will not be spared the wrath of the runners.

There have been several races where I crossed the finish line and did not get my expected award: in the Northern Central Trails Marathon in Maryland I was given a cheap glass mug, which was also the reward handed out one year at the Houston Marathon. The race director in Virginia Beach was even stingier; there, I was only given a finisher's certificate. Although I never uttered a word about it—at least, not to race officials—someone clearly did, because most of these races now offer finisher's medals. In fact, race directors now go above and beyond the call of duty, offering finisher's medals that are getting ever bigger, shinier, and gaudier. Proof once more that it's possible to have too much of a good thing.

Medals have now become so popular that many races of less than marathon distance award them to their participants. Nestled in my collection are medals from the World's Best 10K in San Blas, Puerto Rico, the Amish Country Half-Marathon, the New York City Road Runners New Year's Eve Midnight 5K run, and the Virginia Beach Rock 'N Roll Half-Marathon. I had run each of these races as hard as I could, and felt that I had earned each medal, and yet something was not quite right about receiving that hardware. Perhaps I had become a snob, but I felt that only races of marathon distance or more ought to award medals.

Eventually, the question came up of what to do with them. Originally, an ordinary nail in the wall was good enough to hang them on. I graduated to a bigger nail, and then a hanging display rack I picked up in a yard sale, designed to hold baseball caps. Finally, I just dumped them all into a cabinet drawer.

Packing them away, I found myself rating them. My Boston Marathon medals were my favorite, each one a symbol of high achievement. They knew their value too; no shiny gilded affairs, these. The

Boston Athletic Association opts for pewter, with its emblem, a unicorn, in relief on the front. It's the marathoning equivalent of a pinstripe suit.

In contrast was the playfulness of the Disneyworld Marathon medal. It was an oval with two smaller ovals affixed at the top, giving an approximation of that famous mouse's head. On the face of the medal was a likeness of Mickey himself, tearing down the road in singlet, shorts, and running shoes. The Las Vegas Marathon medal is in the shape of a roulette wheel, appropriately enough. I've also got a ceramic medal, and even an embroidered one.

The ribbons on which the medals were attached reflect each race's personality as well. Their colors range from black to purple, white, green, red, and orange, and in combinations from traditional red, white, and blue to all the colors of the rainbow. The ribbon for the Marine Corps Marathon medals are red and gold, the colors of the Corps, while the Honolulu Marathon medal came on a string of puka shells, and the New Orleans Marathon medal hangs from a string of Mardi Gras beads.

And then there were the shirts. For some reason, most races have traditionally distributed T-shirts bearing a race logo to all race participants. Early on, they were all cotton, but now most races provide technical racing shirts instead. It might be a good way to tell the world that you had done something extraordinary, and it's certainly a good way for a race and its sponsors to get some cheap promotion, but at some point, enough is enough. Every year or so I've had to cull less desirable shirts from the herd, setting them aside for donation to a local homeless shelter.

But there is another kind of memento that I covet, the ultimate kind of racing hardware: an actual award. After I had finished my first marathon, my father was very proud of me. By the time I finished my second one, though, he asked when I would win one. Win? Not likely, I told him. I was a good runner, and usually finished in the top 10 percent of most race fields, but the difference between being good and being elite is huge. As I explained, if I was rested and warmed up at mile 25 and jumped into the race with the members of the elite pack, who had already been running for 2 hours or so, they would easily blow right past me and leave me in the dust. I hated to disappoint Dad, but I told him that I would *never* win a marathon. Simple as that. Just finishing was an accomplishment in itself, and running as hard as I could every time was my victory.

Of course, that didn't mean I couldn't dream a little. I didn't expect to win any races outright, but just placing in my age group would be nice. I achieved a little recognition in a race at Dewey Beach, Delaware one year. It was a 10-mile race with an interesting side competition called the Pump 'n Run. Race volunteers weighed participants, and then loaded up a bench press—full body weight for men, two-thirds of body weight for women—and participants benched this amount as many times as they could shortly before running the race. One minute was then deducted from their finishing time for every repetition they were able to do on the bench.

I signed up for the Pump 'n Run, and bench-pressed my body weight twenty-one times. I then went out and ran a strong race. When it was all over, I discovered that I had won my age group. It was my first award, and even though all I received was a commemorative T-shirt—another T-shirt, for cryin' out loud!—I enjoyed hearing my name being announced, and taking those few but glorious steps forward to claim my prize.

I wasn't completely surprised by my little victory, though. Back in high school I had enjoyed lifting weights with my friends, and I had never given that up, even as I took up running. I might not have been the fastest runner or the strongest lifter, but I can run very fast for a weight lifter, and I am very strong for a runner. The Pump 'n Run rewarded this kind of balanced fitness, and I appreciated that.

But still, I had not won an award for being the fastest runner on race day. My trophy cabinet was still bare.

Then came the Hog Eye Marathon in Fayetteville, Arkansas. Marathon number 85. The night before the race, my friends and I went to a famous local steak joint, Doe's. Supposedly it had been a favorite eating spot for the press corps who followed Bill Clinton on his campaign tours.

They serve two kinds of steak in Doe's: one-pound and two-pound. I showed restraint and ordered the one-pound. It was as good as word of mouth had said it would be. I knew that come race time, the steak would still be with me, like bag of wet cement in my gut. But I wanted to enjoy this time and place with my friends, and one never knows when such a moment may come around again. After eighty-four marathons, I bet that my body would find a way to handle it.

The next morning, though, I worried less about that steak than about the driving rain and wind outside. At the sound of the starter's gun, I set out with several hundred other runners on a very hilly out-and-back course. There is something about truly horrible conditions that focuses the mind, and soon I found myself enjoying the challenge in a crazy kind of way. I wouldn't be out running a marathon in the first place if I didn't like a challenge, and the weather was just one more obstacle to conquer. I gritted my teeth and ran on.

Eventually, the course led us back to town square and the finish line. I collected my medal and then lingered indoors to warm up and have something to eat. When the race results were posted on the wall, I went to check my official time and discovered that I had finished second in my age group. I was going to win an award!

I'm embarrassed to say how excited I was. Dad passed away in 1989, but if he were still alive, I know that he would be thrilled that I had finally won something, even if it took me 85 marathons to do it. My award was a hand-made ceramic plaque, with the race name and logo drawn into it. Aesthetically, it's not much, but to me, it's beautiful.

Looking at all my racing hardware, I'm reminded not only of my years of marathon running, but also of one of my great fears for the future: that some day, all of these medals—and my few awards—will be in a box at a yard sale somewhere, three for a dollar. As I handled some of my medals, I noticed that some of them had already started to corrode. I realized that I didn't have to worry about that far-off yard sale; apparently, my medals wouldn't even last long enough to make it there. What if they all disintegrated little by little? Or what if they were lost in a fire? What was I without my medals?

I knew that if all my medals disappeared, I would feel the loss of the tangible proof that I had led a runner's life. But I realized, too, that they didn't really matter that much. With or without them, I knew what I had achieved. Truth be told, I hardly ever look at any of them anyway; they are to me like the gold in Fort Knox, more of an idea than a physical presence in my day-to-day life. I ran the marathon to discover the depths of my own determination and perseverance. I didn't need a medal to tell me who I was.

Meanwhile, I had other things on my mind that summer. It was June 2004, and Stephanie and I were about to be wed. Even we were surprised at how quickly our relationship had moved along, but though we had dated a little more than one year, we had known each other since we were twelve, so we really felt like we had known each other all our lives, which was more or less true. It was as if we were each getting to know someone we were already very well acquainted with. We had shared history, yet separate lives; wonderful and varied life experiences, yet the same background. As we liked to say to each other, it just made sense.

On the morning of our wedding I woke up early and went for a run—no better way to burn off some of the jitters I felt. I showered and dressed, and drove down from our hotel to the site we had picked: a castle nestled in the Hudson Valley in upstate New York. I marveled that so far, things were going perfectly. Just as that thought went through my mind—hanging there, like a thought balloon in a comic strip—someone asked me if I had the rings on me. I froze. They were still back in my hotel room. Oh, crap. Crap, crap, crap. Un-freakin'-believable.

I jumped in my car and raced the five miles back to the hotel, cruising through stop signs and red lights, almost hoping that a cop would stop me so that I could explain my dilemma and get a police escort. That didn't happen, but I did make it back to the chapel in time, and the ceremony went off without a hitch. After the reception, husband and wife made it back to the hotel room, exhausted but very happy. We celebrated by opening a bottle of '93 Château Lafite Rothschild I had brought back from Médoc. Despite the shaky start, it turned out to be a wonderful day.

The first thing people now want to know about Stephanie was whether she was a marathoner. The answer is no. At first, Stephanie was concerned that I might pressure her into running a marathon, but I told her I could care less whether she ever ran one, and I meant it. Sure, it would be great fun for me to run a marathon next to my wife, but I didn't marry her in order to fulfill that dream; I married her because I love her for who she is, not for what she might become.

Still, Stephanie is very fit. She's a bit of a gym rat, really, which is important to me because I want to be with someone healthy, someone who I can grow old with, someone who can still see life as a great adventure well into our senior years. But run a marathon? Nah. There's plenty of stuff I have no interest in doing. Bungee jumping, for example. I have absolutely zero interest in that.

If Stephanie were to tell me that she didn't think she *could* do it, though, that would be different. Running has taught me to not automatically accept limitations, whether imagined or imposed by others. I don't believe anyone should automatically expect and accept failure, especially not in regard to the marathon. Finishing a marathon is within the reach of anyone with the determination and courage to *just try*.

When we first started dating, Stephanie actually did show some interest in trying to run. Her plan was to run as far as she could and see how that felt. I saved her the suspense and gave her an immediate answer: if she ran for as long as she could, she would only guarantee that she would be tired and miserable when she finally stopped.

Over the years, I've seen the same pattern among people who hate running: when they gave it a shot, they almost always went too far or too fast. The trick, I told her, it to not run until you're exhausted—leave that for the marathons! Instead, I told her to run until she felt fatigued but comfortable at the end. If she didn't want to hate running, she'd need to keep it manageable.

And that's what she did. She began with some walking and easy running on the treadmill, and little by little she worked her way up to running for a half hour straight. In time, she stretched it to an hour.

In November 2003, we took our vacation in New Zealand, which we found to be a magical, wonderful place, filled with beaches, gorges, smoldering thermal springs, and breathtaking mountain ranges. The Kiwis don't take any of this for granted; I'd read that if there's a dangerous, difficult, thrilling way of getting from one point to another, they do it. Naturally, I thought, there must be a marathon. Sure enough, there was, right in the capital city of Auckland, along with a 10K race. I signed up for the marathon, and with my encouragement, Stephanie signed up for the 10K. It was the first race she'd ever entered.

On race morning, I set out before dawn to get to the ferry that brought the marathoners across the harbor to the starting line. It was a beautiful course: almost pretty enough to keep me from cursing the brutal headwind I ran against over the last few miles of the race. As I neared the finish line, I wondered how Stephanie had done.

The race finished in a park, and it didn't take me long to spot her across the open field. As I waved to her, I ticked off items on my mental triage checklist: she was upright, she was walking, and she was smiling. When I got to her, I gave her a big kiss and asked how it went.

"Great," she said. "I finished in just under an hour."

"That's a great time," I told her. "You should be proud."

"Yeah, I am," she told me. "But around mile four, I thought, *Well, wouldn't a cup of coffee and a newspaper be nice right now?*"

So, there might be no marathon run together for us. Or maybe there will be. Either way, it's okay; Stephanie had proven—as much to herself as to me—that she could run one if she wanted to. But running isn't her passion, it's mine. Her passion is for art, both as a painter and a teacher. I love that she has such strong opinions, dedication, knowledge, and talent for it. That kind of passion is, to me, the fullest embodiment of what is best in our nature. Our appreciation for each other's passion is more important to us than being able to fully share in the object of each other's joy. We each feel deeply about something, and are willing to risk something of ourselves for it. That alone makes us kindred spirits.

We do actually run together sometimes. I think of these runs not just as workouts; they're couple-time, when we share stories or ideas, or just enjoy a break from the rest of the world. Instead of being in competition with our relationship, running has, I think, strengthened it.

After all these years, I think I finally got it right.

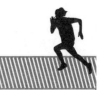

Running Tip #15

How to Do the Thing You Love with the One You Love

Training with your romantic partner is not impossible, but if you want to make it work, it's a good idea to follow some basic guidelines.

- *Put the relationship first.* Running with a mate can be tricky. The key is to not do anything to demean or demoralize your partner. So forget your training schedule. If you push too hard, he or she will get very cranky. The point is to demonstrate what you already know: that running can be fun. Do your hard workout earlier or later in the day, or on another day altogether.
- *Make your run together your entire workout.* Don't use your run together as a portion of a longer workout. That implies that the run was inadequate, which could undermine your mate's confidence. So start and finish together.
- *Make sure your partner has the proper gear.* Chances are your nonrunning mate will show up for your first run together wearing cross-training shoes, a cotton T-shirt, and sweatpants. In other words, all the wrong things. If you think missing your anniversary led to a big fight, see what happens when running with you causes your mate to have chafing and blisters. So go shopping together for proper clothing and good running shoes.

→

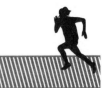

- *Figure out what works for your partner.* It's your job to show your partner a fun time; if he or she enjoys the run, he or she will be back for more.

- *Don't be the boss.* After years of running and racing, it's easy to think we know everything about running. But if you tell your partner what to do, you reduce him or her to an underling. So don't order; create a dialogue instead. He or she will probably follow your advice anyway, but that will be his or her decision. It makes a difference.

- *Don't forget these rules on race day.* When your partner is ready to try a first race, be supportive. Offer to run a race with her or him, at her or his pace. But remember: this is your mate's race, not yours; you're just support crew with a number. If your partner would rather run without you, decide together where you'll meet afterward, and ask what you should bring for after the race.

Good Things Come in Small Packages

My next marathon was only a few weeks after I got married. I met up with Dave in Calgary, Canada, to run a marathon. The race was held in conjunction with the annual Stampede Rodeo—not really a sport that I could identify with. But stranger to me than the idea of roping cattle was the gold band that I fingered on my left hand during the race. I quickly got used to it, though, which I took to be a good sign, and when I crossed the finish line, I received a large western-style belt buckle on a ribbon as a medal, which seemed a fitting memento for that particular race.

That was marathon number 88. When people heard that I'd run that many races, they'd usually ask me which one was my favorite. I didn't know what to say. There were obvious contenders, like New York, Boston, and Paris. I did love them all. But like a child in a candy shop, I just couldn't decide. Finally, I came upon an answer that was honest: my favorite marathon is ... the next one. People smiled, but it was really a dodge, and we all knew it.

Little by little, I started to narrow the field, if not to a particular marathon, then at least to a category. The big races were the ones that people were most familiar with. These behemoths were cities unto

184

themselves, and they were like huge running festivals. They were *events.* But with the bright lights and press coverage came the uglier side. These races were demanding, high maintenance mistresses, requiring one to fight for entry, to battle for hotels and flights, and to wake up early to rush to the starting line to wait with tens of thousands of other runners for the start, and then pick one's way through the crowds at the finish for family and friends, all lost in a sea of sweaty bodies. These races were memorable, but they often seemed like so much *work.*

That said, big-city marathons should not to be missed, and I returned to them again and again. But were they my favorite races? Not necessarily. There was something more important than the flash of the big-city races; I learned to love the allure of the small-town marathon. Modest, unassuming, more friendly and personal, these were the races I truly enjoyed. Still, people didn't seem to completely believe that. I could see it in their eyes. Sure, they seemed to say, that sounds nice, but you'd never turn down the New York Marathon for a race in, say, Idaho, would you?

Wouldn't I? I decided to put it to the test. I needed to add Idaho to my list of states anyway, so Idaho it would be for marathon number 89. The Mesa Falls Marathon in Ashton, to be exact.

First, I had to get there. Whoever said that it's the journey that matters, not the destination, never spent a lot of time waiting around in an airport. As soon as I went online to book my flights for the race, I realized that things would not be as simple as I expected. There weren't any direct flights from D.C. to Ashton, and among the circuitous routes that were available, there were precious few options.

But that was okay; I hadn't expected booking my flights to be a run in the park. Ultimately, the ones I chose would land me in Idaho well past sunset on the day before the race. No problem. I could handle that, too. There was no commercial airport in Ashton, which meant that I would have to rent a car in Idaho Falls and drive an hour to get to my destination. Still not a problem; I've had to do that before in other big-city races. I would miss the prerace pasta dinner and all the camaraderie that's usually found there, but that wasn't the end of the world, since there would be plenty of time to meet people on the course during the race.

After spending nearly the entire day outbound waiting for flights and making connections, I finally arrived in Idaho Falls. It was a tiny airport, but that was a good thing, since there was no need to take a shuttle to an off-site baggage claim area: I could just step down onto the tarmac, walk into the terminal, get my rental car and go. Except that despite having made a reservation, no one was available at the off-site office to set me up with a car. Quicker than I could say "grrrrrrrr," though, I rented another car from a friendly young woman at a competitor's sales desk, and was soon on my way to Ashton. Still, none of these transportation problems would have happened in Boston, Chicago, or New York. Advantage: big-city marathon.

An hour later, I was driving down ID-47 in Ashton, Idaho, also known more simply as Main Street. I was glad for the sign postings, because I easily could have missed it. With a population of 1,129, there wasn't going to be a lot of street life anyway, especially not around midnight, which is when I arrived. The marathon Web site had listed available lodging, and I opted for the Four Seasons Motel, which was said to be near where the runners were to line up for transport to the starting line on race morning. When booking the room a few weeks earlier over the phone, the clerk told me almost apologetically that the price would be $45 per night. I magnanimously told him that would be perfectly fine. As I edged down Main Street in the quiet darkness, I discovered it on my right, one of those wayside-type inns with parking spots in front of each room. There was a note affixed to the front door of the office addressed to me, letting me know which room was mine, and that it had been left open for me. This would NEVER happen in New York. Not on marathon weekend, not ever. Not even anywhere within 100 miles of

New York. I smiled with relief; at this hour, every moment was precious, and the sooner I could lay my head on a pillow, the better.

I ambled over to my room, swung the door open and found ... pretty much just a room. It was nothing fancy, but it was certainly serviceable. A clean bed, a TV, and hot and cold running water. Gazing out the door, I realized that the local high school's parking lot, where we would board buses for transport to the race start, was literally right across the street. At least I could sleep to the very last moment, and needed only to make sure I had all my running gear on as I stumbled out the door.

The alarm woke me from a deep slumber, and I looked out the window. Still dark outside. Nothing unusual, since many races have a predawn starting time. There were already two school buses idling in the parking lot, with a handful of runners milling about. Only eleven racers participated in the race's inaugural running in 1997, and the field ballooned to forty the following year.

From what I could see while peering out that window, it hadn't grown very much since then. There were only a few hundred runners, apparently no media representatives whatsoever, and precious few spectators. Still, I don't think I'd ever before had such a comforting prerace moment. I'd had some close calls in the past getting to the starting line in time, but this would not be one of those days.

Fifteen minutes later, while identifying constellations in the clear sky, I walked up to the folding table that served as headquarters for race-day packet pickup. The temperature was in the upper 30s, although warmer weather was predicted for later in the day. Race Director Dave Jacobson checked my name off the list and handed me my packet and a smart-looking polo shirt with an embroidered race logo. "You," Dave told me, "are the first person from Washington, D.C., to run the Mesa Falls Marathon." That meant I would hold the course record for a D.C. marathoner just by crossing the finish line. I began imagining my press release as I trotted back across the street to my motel room to drop off my shirt and goody bag.

Climbing aboard one of the buses minutes later, I peered toward the back for the one thing worth its weight in gold to a runner before a race: a bathroom. There it was, tucked away in the corner. Breathing a sigh of relief, I settled into one of the plush seats, felt the warmth flowing upward from the bus's heaters, and unwrapped my personal "breakfast of champions": two energy bars and a sports drink.

The bus was buzzing with conversation, and soon I met all the runners seated around me. There was a father-daughter team, and quite a few out-of-town runners. As it turned out, though, no one had traveled as far as I did. More than one person wore confused expressions when they found out where I was from; they seemed to find it hard to believe that anyone would come so far for such a small race.

As I sat talking with my new neighbors, I realized that very few of them were first-time marathoners. In fact, several of the runners had already completed over 100, and one runner had completed over 200. Apparently, I was no longer the craziest person in the room. This highlighted a characteristic of smaller races that I soon came to appreciate; the average depth of experience among the participants in small marathons seemed to be vastly greater than that of the people to be found in the typical big city marathon. This meant that I'd be able to tap into the collective running wisdom of this group throughout the day about various other marathons, and, more importantly, get valuable information about the marathon course from people who had run this race before. As the bus pulled out of the parking lot for the 45-minute ride to the race start, I fell into a light sleep.

The bus groaned through a turn, and my eyes fluttered open. The sky was slowly beginning to brighten, and the bus, having left the highway, was coming to a stop next to, well, next to nothing, really. We were in the middle of nowhere. There was no building or man-made structure to be seen anywhere, apart from the road we drove in on. I didn't know it at the time, but we were in Targhee National Forest, by the Island Park caldera. We were at an altitude of 6,142 feet, roughly one mile above sea level.

The air felt crisp and clean as I left the bus and moved toward the impromptu starting line along with the rest of the runners. In New York, sheer luck gets you close to the front of the pack; in Boston, it's proven speed. In the Mesa Falls Marathon, however, all you need to do is step forward and pick your spot.

I chose to stand behind some of the faster-looking runners; close enough to feel the excitement of seeing open road ahead when the race begins, but not so close as to give myself illusions of being an elite racer. Dave Jacobson led us through the traditional prerace remarks, and then, without fanfare, sent us off.

This small phalanx of runners moved briskly along the asphalt as snippets of conversation broke out here and there among us. At that altitude, I knew I would be laboring to maintain my usual pace, so I tried to rein in my legs, which were feeling particularly springy. The course would eventually bring us down to an elevation of 5,260 feet, for a net drop of 882 feet, so I wasn't worried about a slow start; I would have plenty of opportunity to pick up the pace later on.

I followed the pack through a left turn, and found myself on a wide dirt road, heading deeper into the wilderness. Full daybreak was upon us now, revealing rolling hills on both sides of the road, covered in brush and short trees. Up ahead, I was told, there would be wonderful views of the Grand Teton mountain range. One thing I knew not to expect, though, were spectators cheering us on in the coming miles, but with all of the great scenery around me, I was starting to think that they might not be missed.

It was at that moment that I realized we were not quite as alone as I thought. Strange noises echoed from distance. There were wild animals out there howling at us. Another runner then told me that he had seen a moose in the first mile of the race. Despite its great size, the beast disappeared soundlessly into the brush. These other animals, however, did not seem quite as shy. A volunteer at mile 8 told me that coyotes and wolves had given him the eye as he set up our refreshments earlier in the morning. I felt an instinctual moment of panic, but then I realized that these animals were probably more afraid of us than we were of them. As long as I didn't drift so far back of the pack that I'd seem separated from the herd, I knew I'd be safe. Just as I relaxed, the howling subsided, as if on cue.

Just then the Tetons came into view, bathed in bright morning sunlight. They were indeed magnificent, even if we were too far away to fully appreciate their sculpted beauty. Then the fickle road turned us away from this sight and plunged us into the woods. We were led onto a bike path, which emptied onto a small scenic overlook. Hundreds of feet below us and perhaps a half-mile away, the Snake River plunged off what appeared to be a wide, stone tabletop. It was the race's namesake, the Lower Mesa Falls. I paused a moment to fully take in the beautiful view. Reluctantly, I turned away and followed the race path back into the woods.

It was about this time that I fell into a conversation with Matt, whose race turned out to be a family effort. Matt's sisters and cousins were providing vehicular support—"support" in the sense of screaming and yelling from an open van door during a slow drive-by.

"Know those folks?" I joked.

"Yeah," he admitted sheepishly. "My brother and cousin are out here also somewhere, running their first marathon."

Matt already had a little marathon experience, having run the Roxbury (Idaho) Marathon. "Now *that's* a small race," he told me. "Just twenty-two runners." I guess he entered the Mesa Falls Marathon to see what it would be like to do a big race.

At mile 13 we came to a short stretch of paved road that led us to Bear Claw Junction, which was the starting point for the half-marathoners. Some marathon runners don't like having fresh legs suddenly thrown in alongside them at a race's mid-point, since it can throw off their pacing. As for me, on that day at least, I was glad to have a little more company as we descended into the brush and found ourselves once again on a dirt trail.

The path on which we were now running was narrower than the road on which we had started, but it soon revealed itself as one of the most scenic stretches of any marathon I've ever run—four beautiful miles along Idaho's Warm River. Our trail was halfway up the side of a valley, providing commanding views of the river below and the valley around us. The weather had warmed, the sun was shining, the trees and bushes were lush and green, and the river was an inviting blue. Matt told me that there was no truth to the river's name, however; the Warm River was frigid this time of year. No matter; it *looked* inviting. I found myself gliding along the path, lost in runner's nirvana. I told Matt that even though this was just his second marathon, nature and the race director had conspired to give him a grand treat. He would see many wonderful scenes if he continued racing, but there might never be another moment as perfect as this one.

And suddenly it was gone. We came off the trail and returned to asphalt roads, rolling through rich Idaho farmland. The views here were less spectacular, but no less interesting, at least for this city boy. I had been warned by several runners, though, that there would be a big hill coming up shortly at about mile 18, so I girded myself for the worst. There was a hill all right, but it was not a heartbreaker, not in the Boston mold. I threw my mental lasso around the runner in front of me—fitting imagery for this part of the country—and labored up to the crest. With the hill now behind me, I settled in to a steady pace and started to think more about the finish line.

Houses multiplied alongside the road, farmland gave way to stores and short buildings, and I realized that I was on the outskirts of Ashton and nearing the finish line. The streets were quiet as I passed an auto parts store and a thrift shop. Up ahead on my right were grain silos, and I knew the end was at hand. There were some spectators cheering now, as a volunteer steered us through a right turn, and toward Ashton City Park.

As I crossed the finish line, I heard my name being announced—always a nice touch—and was awarded a finisher's medal. Marathon number 89 was over.

But things would soon get even better. Our goody bags contained a coupon, redeemable after the race, for a huckleberry shake from City Drug. I retrieved the coupon and set off for my hard-earned treat. Along the way I passed other runners who had already claimed their prize, and their smiles quickened my step.

City Drug was only a few short blocks away, but it was of another time and place. It was a small storefront shop, featuring a soda counter with stools. An older woman gave me a smile as I came in, and a young boy reached down below the counter and produced a genuine, prepoured huckleberry shake. I didn't even have to say a word; it must have been pretty obvious why I was there.

Stepping out into the street, I took a long pull on the straw, savoring the creamy coolness. As I walked back to the park, I shouted encouragement to the other runners nearing the finish line—"Get the shake! Get the shake!" Back at the park I found the race director, Dave, and thanked him for a top-notch marathon. The last runners were still more than an hour away from finishing—there would be 120 finishers in all—but Dave was already looking to the future. Heady with success, he was hoping to expand the race. "We can accommodate about 500 runners before we have to have any restrictions," he said. It sounded like an explosion of runners, but it would still just amount to a small 5K field back home.

I picked an inviting patch of sun-warmed grass near the covered picnic area and settled down for the awards ceremony. The winning times were 2:51:12 for the men, and 3:12:27 for the women. Very respectable times, but far from the otherworldly ones posted by the world's elite runners at the big races. My own finishing time left me well behind the leaders, but as I watched them claim their prizes, I felt that we were at least still members of the same species.

As the winners of the various age categories were honored, and random prizes distributed—everything from a heart rate monitor to beef jerky—I realized that many of these people knew each other, and had probably known each other for years. The camaraderie among them was palpable. I found myself daydreaming of having lived here, trained here, and raced here, so I could share in their jokes and stories.

Finally, all the awards had been claimed, all the prizes had been distributed, and it was time to go. I showered, gathered my things, and checked out of the Four Seasons Motel, saying good-bye to the owner's young son, who was manning the front desk. I drove back to Little Falls, dropped off the car, and boarded my flight.

Gazing out the window past the thin, wispy clouds to the farmland far below, I thought about the Mesa Falls Marathon, and the other small towns I had visited for marathons. Tupelo, Mississippi. Fayetteville, Arkansas. Tulsa, Oklahoma. And Wichita, Kansas, so quiet on a Saturday night downtown that I wouldn't have been surprised if the city rolled up their sidewalks after dark. These races all felt like family gatherings, with people working hard to make the events come off smoothly, for no glory other than to have managed to make it happen and to have shown a few hundred runners a good time.

Sometimes, though, things didn't go quite so well, like in Louisville, Kentucky, where a mismeasured course added an unnecessary mile to the race, leaving runners swarming like angry bees at the finish line. There were times when the aid stations were not well-stocked, when there were so few spectators and fellow runners that it seemed to be a race in theory only. But still, there was something to these races, an earnestness that seemed truer to the marathoning spirit than the marketing and spectacle of the big city races. And those huckleberry shakes, of course.

But would I really trade Ashton for the New York City Marathon? No. What is lost in numbers is gained in excitement; there is no phenomenon as startling as the sight of a huge mass of people running down the street, not in panic, but with joy and determination. But if I had only experienced the Big Race, I would not have a complete understanding of the marathon.

So, my favorite marathon? I still can't tell you. Perhaps I'm too greedy. I want them all.

Soon after returning from Idaho, I had another interesting running adventure in my own backyard. In the green spaces throughout Washington, D.C., creatures stirred, awakening from their seventeen-year slumber. Soon, they would arise in the thousands from their underground lairs, like graveyard zombies, and invade the city, filling the air with a hellishly loud buzz. They were short and squat with thick, greenish bodies and blood-red eyes, and they were called "Brood X." The city seemed transfixed in nervous anticipation, but was powerless to stop them.

Despite their ominous name and hellish appearance, they were, in fact, just insects. Cicadas. And rather than being worried about them, most people seemed intrigued. As zero-hour drew near, the local newspapers themselves became infested with articles about them. We were told where we could expect the highest concentrations, and how to protect trees with netting. There were even recipes on how to prepare them for dinner. But no one told runners what they could expect.

The days flew by, and every morning I stepped outside, only to find … nothing. As it turned out, not every neighborhood would get a visit from the Brood. Why were they snubbing me? This was expected to be a seminal D.C. event, and I wasn't invited to the party.

I realized that if I wanted to experience these pests, I would actually have to go looking for them. I had read that areas farther northwest that had older trees would be harder hit by the little buggers. So I laced up my running shoes, corralled a running partner, and went north, entering Rock Creek Park near the Carter Baron amphitheater.

We soon came across our quarry. We saw first one, then another cicada laid out on the ground in front of us. There were dozens more nearby. Then we saw one fly right into a parked car. It occurred to me that was the equivalent of failing to notice a skyscraper and walking into it facefirst. These were not bright creatures. We continued our run.

I soon became accustomed to seeing small black clumps whizzing around us. Their style of flying can best described as awkward and clumsy, even out of control. I wondered if perhaps they were screaming in panic as they flew past. Suddenly, a cicada dove straight at me. I ducked to avoid a head-on collision. I looked over to see my running partner twisting and pirouetting herself to avoid contact. It was then that we stopped viewing the cicadas as silly little aerial clowns and more as incoming missiles, and we began to wonder how much a direct hit from one would sting. Luckily, we made it home with that question still unanswered.

A few days later I ran a different route up near Glover Park. Hurtling down Massachusetts Avenue, I saw hundreds of little black corpses on the sidewalk. Revulsion soon tuned to curiosity, which turned to sadness. Seventeen years of waiting, for only a few days of life. Their silly little existence suddenly seemed more precious, making my own life that much more valuable, too. Their ungainly attempts at flight now reminded me of so many runners who trump their own clumsiness with sheer determination, and who, through their efforts, gain a type of grace.

The cicadas no longer seemed to me to be tiny invaders, but instead, in a way, little creatures with whom I could share a strange kinship. Not born myself with a natural runner's body or a smooth stride, I run fearlessly, just like the cicadas seem to fly, knowing that honest sweat has its own grace, and knowing, too, that my days here are numbered. Perhaps we weren't so very different after all.

Of course, my empathy has its limits. If ever I run into the wall of an office building by accident, I'm hanging up my running shoes for good.

Running Tip #16

Mind Games

- *Stay mindful of what you're doing.* It's like driving: you don't have to hold the steering wheel in a death grip, but you should be calmly aware of both your car and your surroundings.
- *Have a checklist.* Are you landing too heavily? Are you swinging your arms too far? How's your breathing? How's your posture? Become aware of your bad tendencies, and keep an eye out for them.
- *Manage your intensity.* Some runners visualize how strong they'll feel at specific, difficult parts of an upcoming race. Others repeat a supportive phrase like a mantra. I like to visualize catastrophe. It's actually not as crazy as it sounds. If I can accept the worst that could happen on race day, I've conquered my fears, and I can relax and just run. Find out what works for you. Your mind is a puzzle that can be solved, and once you find the right answer, you can achieve your best times.

There and Back:
Adventures in South Africa

I sat in the dark theater, gazing up at the image on the screen. It was of a man pumping his arms rhythmically as he ran over brown, unpaved earth. The man was Haile Gebrselassie, the great Ethiopian middle-distance runner, and the movie was *Endurance,* the film that chronicled his rise from poverty in Ethiopia to Olympic gold in Atlanta. The opening scene was of Gebrselassie on a training run, covering the African countryside with long, powerful strides, gliding over rocks and hills with no display of effort. He looked like a running god, and the land looked primeval. This, to me, was Africa.

But Africa was also a land of war, oppression, corruption, and disease. Alongside its great beauty sat great hardship. It was difficult for my mind to encompass the whole of it. I've often imagined the world as being crisscrossed with running trails, interrupted here and there by mountains and oceans. Some of them are paved and measured. Most are not. Some haven't even been discovered yet. But try as might, I couldn't quite fit Africa into my vision of the world; I couldn't imagine racing there.

Clearly, something needed to be done. Stephanie, always up for a good adventure, agreed. I went online, signed up for the Two Oceans Marathon, to take place on March 26, 2005, and booked our trip to South Africa. One way or the other, I was going to sort this out.

Our itinerary would be challenging. We were to fly to Johannesburg, then on to Hoedspruit for a safari, and then down to Cape Town, where the race would be held. All that sounded fine, except that our return flight was booked for the afternoon of race day. Not an ideal plan, but that was the only schedule that met all of the conflicting requirements of our work lives and the available flights and excursions, so that was the way it was going to be. If nothing else, the fear of missing an international flight would be a great incentive to run faster.

The conceit of our age is that we live in a world that is becoming ever smaller. Interconnected economies, e-mail and online services, and fast, relatively cheap flights make almost any part of the globe as close as your next-door neighbor.

Don't you believe it. Africa is still a long way from the United States. From our home in D.C., we made our way to New York for a flight to Johannesburg, with a layover in Dakar, Senegal. The entire adventure would require almost a full twenty-four hours, but instead of moaning about the discomfort of it all, I actually appreciated the difficulty involved. Something magical happens during a long flight to a distant, exotic land. The idea of adventure ferments in your mind until it is fully risen upon arrival, making you hungry for whatever you may discover. This process takes time, and as we boarded our flight at JFK airport, I knew we would have all the time we needed.

That was the emotional argument in favor of a long flight. The physical arguments weighed in against it. I tossed and turned in my seat, bent and straightened my legs in a futile attempt to find a truly comfortable position, all to no avail. There were some bright spots, though; plenty of good movies to watch, and one truly memorable sight—a predawn liftoff from Dakar, with a view of dozens of fishermen slowly heading out to sea in their small boats, hundreds of feet below us, as the dark blue of the sky bled crimson and orange. It was an impossibly beautiful moment. I settled in for the remainder of the flight, contemplating Africa.

Eight hours later, the sun was setting as we touched down in Johannesburg. We would be spending only one short night there before leaving first thing in the morning for another flight to Hoedspruit. As we drove from the airport to our hotel on the edge of town, any guilt I felt about not spending more time in Johannesburg was allayed by our driver, who, while insisting that security was improving downtown, warned us about the prolific and violent street crime. When apartheid ended and movement by nonwhites was no longer restricted, millions of people migrated to the cities with a dream of finding a better job. When those jobs did not materialize, the dispossessed survived as best they could, building shantytowns on the fringes of the city, and, in some cases, preying on those around them. Our driver said that some downtown hotels had closed because of the crime, to which the government responded by installing street cameras.

During the ride, our driver taught us a few basic words of Zulu, one of the nine African languages spoken throughout the country. Most South Africans speak several languages in addition to Afrikaans and English, including Zulu. It was very humbling. Like many Americans, I'm limited to English and a smattering of high school Spanish. Stephanie and I were entranced as he ran through several dialects, occasionally making clucking sounds that no Westerner could emulate. As we drove past some abandoned buildings and gold mines, I wondered at this unique place. *Egoli*, the Zulu name for Johannesburg—City of Gold.

In the morning I made use of the treadmill in our hotel for a quick run, not wanting to get lost on the city streets. On the television was Nelson Mandela, who, even in retirement, is generally looked upon as perhaps the world's foremost moral authority. He was onstage at a concert on Human Rights Day, the national holiday memorializing the murder of sixty-nine pepole in the 1960 Sharpeville massacre. Taking the stage after a performance by Annie Lennox, Mandela said that healthy women were also victims of the AIDS epidemic. AIDS was becoming a disaster of epic proportions in South Africa, fueled by misconceptions about its origin and how to cure it. Some South Africans even believe that the virus can be cured by sleeping with virgins. The day after Mandela's speech, the local newspapers reported that a man with AIDS was arrested for brutally killing his wife, his wife's child, and his wife's mother because his wife stopped sleeping with him.

A few hours later, Stephanie and I boarded a small plane bound for Hoedspruit. After our long journey the day before, we were happy that this flight would only last a single hour. As the plane descended, I nervously scanned the countryside for signs of an airport, but found none. Nevertheless, the plane continued to drop, and then we touched down.

Stepping out into the bright sunshine, I was struck by the unlikeliness of the place. The airport was a tiny military airstrip that was converted to civilian use. The terminal consisted only of a small building outfitted with a couch, several comfortable chairs, and animal prints on the walls. It looked like a room in which you might relax with a drink after a long day traversing the grassy veldt.

After collecting our bags, we stepped through the building to our transport, and immediately saw a waterbuck—a deer-like animal—leap across the road into the bush. We weren't even off the airport grounds and we'd had our first wild animal sighting. This was the Africa of our dreams.

The wildlife preserves of Hoedspruit are large, but not the endless open miles of our imaginations. Fences—some of them electrified—separated the various preserves. These areas are large enough to get lost in, and for even the largest animals to hide. With the beautiful Drakensberg Mountains as a backdrop, we made our way to our campsite within the

Gwalagwala game preserve. This was nothing like the scouting adventures of my youth. These tents are mounted on large wooden platforms, and enclose modern accommodations, including a bed, proper bathroom, and electricity. There was also a treehouse bar in which to meet other travelers, and an open-air dining area.

Our hosts were Dorian and Ann, a couple who had decided later in life that they wanted a change, and gambled on buying untilled farmland and converting it into a game preserve. It soon became apparent, however, that they were still trying to figure out their proper place in this environment. Ann had unwittingly managed to adopt several animals, including a young, wayward warthog, despite concerns that it might not be good for a wild animal to become too accustomed to being in close quarters with humans. Still, the little warthog had a certain charm, and it was fun watching him try to chew the elastic laces on my running shoes. He pulled back the laces several times, only to jump with a start when it snapped out of his mouth. After several attempts, he grunted and turned away, much to our amusement.

After settling in and having lunch, we set out for an afternoon game ride. Early mornings and late afternoons are the best times for viewing animals, when the sun is the least oppressive and the animals are more active. *Not unlike runners,* I thought, as we clambered in to the open Land Rover.

We had scheduled three game rides over the next several days, in search of the African safari Holy Grail—sightings of the Big Five: lion, rhino, elephant, water buffalo, and leopard. We managed to see all except the elusive leopard, and saw many others as well, including giraffe, hyena, cheetah, and impala.

The impala were perhaps the most memorable, leaping as if staying planted on the earth took more effort than getting airborne. Locals referred to the impala as their "McDonald's," which had nothing to do with fast food, but instead refers to the pattern made by the distinctive black streaks running down each of their haunches and their tails, creating nature's version of the Golden Arches.

I wondered what it would be like to have so much power in my legs, to be able to leap so quickly and gracefully. Watching wild animals filled me with a sense of awe, and also revealed the limitations of my own body. Humans are not the fastest, strongest, or most graceful creatures found in nature, and I could only imagine how pitiful even the fastest among us must look to the rest of the animal kingdom. I recalled reading, however, that humans can track and run down game on foot over long distances, due in large part to the amazing shock-absorbing properties of our feet. We might not be the fastest, but as long as we can keep the game in sight, we can eventually overtake it, like the proverbial tortoise beating the hare.

This all reminded me of some trash talk I had recently engaged in with a friend at a local gym. He was younger than I, very fit and athletic, and had just started running. He boasted that he was already a faster runner than I was. I assured him that I could beat him. He told me that he was faster than I was in the 5K. I told him that might be true, but I'd race him in a 10K. He said he could still beat me at that distance. Maybe so, I replied, but if it took a half-marathon, a marathon, or a 50-mile ultramarathon, I would eventually beat him. I could run all those races, and I would eventually win. He was silent after that.

Not everyone among our group seemed enamored with the aesthetic beauty of the animals in quite the same way. One great big strapping fellow—a former rugby player—seemed to look at nature as one big all-you-can-eat smorgasbord. He talked a great deal about the South African taste for meat. From wild buck—especially one type called "kudu"—to crocodile and ostrich, South Africans will eat it all, as long as it once moved. They are carnivores with a capital "C." My wife is no vegetarian, but she was astounded. "Don't you ever eat any salad?" she asked. Winking, our companion said, "When we want vegetables, we eat chicken." I suddenly wondered whether a prerace carb load might be harder to find than I thought.

Managing a game preserve isn't all fun, though, as Dorian told me. He pointed to a young giraffe that was limping. His right hind leg was marred by a gaping wound, and his footprints were marked with spots of blood. He had been attacked by a hyena. As we watched the suffering animal, we wanted to help it, but that is not how things are handled on a game preserve. To maintain the balance of things, the animals must be left alone in all but the most extreme circumstances. The hyenas have to eat also, of course. It seemed cruel, but this was nature's way.

At our last evening there, we sat once again under the stars, drinking South African wine, eating a delicious dinner that did, thankfully, include some fresh vegetables, and compared stories with our fellow travelers. Several of them were South Africans on holiday, and they were open about their feelings about their country and recent events. Their mood seemed hopeful, although they had their doubts about particular politicians. Their criticisms seemed reaffirming, though, because not one of them stated any disillusionment with the overall direction their nation had taken over the previous decade, or even with much of what the current administration was trying to achieve.

Eventually the conversation drifted around to my upcoming challenge, and everyone wished me good luck in the race. The Two Oceans Marathon seemed to be quite well known; even people who were not runners were quite familiar with it. Finally, the dessert was over, the last of the wine had been drunk, and it was time for Stephanie and me to get our things together for our flight out the next morning. We would be departing Hoedspruit for Cape Town, and suddenly the race, which had not seemed real before, loomed large.

Cape Town is a beautiful, wondrous city, embodying much of what is best and worst about South Africa. Nestled between the sheltered waters of Table Bay and the majestic heights of Table Mountain, Cape

Town has a long and checkered past. Phoenicians and Arabs thought it had magnetic powers that would draw ships to their doom along its rocky coast, and the Portuguese explorer Vasca da Gama sighted it as he rounded the Cape of Good Hope in 1498. The town was laid out in 1652 by the Dutch East India Company as a replenishment station for its fleet. The local population mostly succumbed to smallpox brought inadvertently by the colonialists, and the surviving indigenous population mostly worked as poorly treated laborers.

In 1795 and 1806, the British invaded South Africa, and by 1843, it had annexed large parts of the country. Clashes with native Zulus and the rising population of Dutch-speaking farmers, known as Boers, led to the Anglo-Boer Wars of 1880–1881 and 1899–1902. The British crushed the Boers with a scorched-earth policy, burning farms and establishing the world's first concentration camps. Eventually, over 136,000 Dutch Afrikaners were imprisoned in these camps, in which more than 26,000 women and children died from typhoid, dysentery, and neglect.

The Union of South Africa was formed in 1910, and the policy of oppression against the native population reached full fruition in 1948 with the creation of apartheid, a complex system that separated the races by law. Apartheid weathered international boycotts and domestic protest and violence, until President F. W. de Klerk unexpectedly abandoned it in 1990, and began negotiating with Nelson Mandela, his formerly jailed adversary. Mandela's African National Congress then won South Africa's first full and open election, and South Africa's journey from darkness was completed when president-elect Mandela announced that "Never, never, and never again shall it be that this beautiful land will again experience the oppression of one by another."

Cape Town reflects all of this history. From its 300-year-old Castle of Good Hope, to its beautiful architecture and manicured gardens, Cape Town shows the best of its colonial past. But then there is District Six, the vibrant port area that was bulldozed in 1979 and declared "whites-only."

Loud protests followed, and the area was kept barren. Today a museum commemorates the destruction of this neighborhood. And there is also Robben Island, an Alcatraz-like penal colony sitting in the bay, where Mandela and others spent years imprisoned for dedicating their lives to fighting apartheid.

Stephanie and I settled into our hotel room overlooking Greenmarket Square, built in 1710 and still used daily as a popular flea market. One evening, we were serenaded by a free jazz concert held there. From our window we could see the square, nearby churches, and the looming mass of Table Mountain, draped in the morning hours with clouds. Over the next several days we would visit all of these sights, riding a cable car to the mountain top, wandering the through towns and visiting museums. Still, my mind kept turning to the marathon.

The Two Oceans Marathon is actually poorly named; it is not a marathon at all. Rather, it is a 56-kilometer ultramarathon, with a half-marathon option also available. The most striking feature of the ultra is its course profile. Starting with a small hill early on, the race meanders over flat roads for the first 28 kilometers, but then it takes a nasty turn as it makes a precipitous ascent of Chapman's Peak at kilometer 34. It then screams back down over the next 6 kilometers, and, at the point when a regular marathon would be over, begins a steep ascent of Constantia Nek. It's the kind of course profile to strike fear even into the heart of an experienced marathoner.

I was concerned about the race, and decided that seeing the beast might allay my fears. Stephanie and I decided to take a tour of the Cape of Good Hope, and the driver readily agreed to drive along as much of the race course for us as he could. Soon, we were driving up to Chapman's Peak, called simply Chappies by the locals. Even in a microbus I could appreciate the steepness of the climb. After severe rock falls plagued the area, the road up Chappies was closed and the course was altered to skirt around Chappies from 2000 to 2004.

I could see why so many runners were disappointed. The view was amazing. The road hugged the pale orange cliff-side, providing a beautiful view of Hout Bay to the west. Our driver pointed out the 1,560 meters of fencing and the concrete canopy that had been installed as part of the new safety measures that allowed the race to return to Chappies in 2004. The netting looked quite fragile to me, though, and I imagined struggling up this road on race day, conquering Chappies, and pausing to celebrate one of the greatest moments of my running life, only to be clunked on the head by a falling boulder. I made a mental note to remember not to pause here on race day if I could help it.

Finally, Stephanie and I found ourselves at the Cape of Good Hope, the storied tip of Africa, where the rough waters of the Atlantic meet the warm waters of the Indian Ocean. We stared out over the open expanse of water before us, and marveled at how far we had come. Ahead of us still was a visit to a penguin colony at Boulders Beach—yet one more sign that we were far, far from home. But standing at the Cape seemed to be the crowning moment. There was, finally, nowhere farther to go.

After feeling like the race would never come, I suddenly found myself picking up my race packet at the University of Cape Town the day before the start. I meandered through the expo, had a pasta dinner in the hotel restaurant, and then settled back in our hotel room with some good reading: the racing instructions. Among the papers included was a booklet entitled "Information and Statistics." It was an absolute compendium of minutiae about the race. There were 7,830 participants registered in the ultra. There were nearly four times as many male ultra runners as female, though there were 339 husband and wife teams. I was disappointed to see that there was no statistic on divorces caused by racing together.

There were also three runners going for their thirtieth finish, and twenty-four runners who would be celebrating their birthday on race day. The oldest registered runner was seventy-six, and the youngest was nineteen. Sixty-three countries were represented, although only 360 runners were from overseas, and only thirty-three were from the United States. I realized then that the worst I could do as a finisher would be to place thirty-third in my category—not bad for bragging rights back home, as long as there were no follow-up questions about the number of runners.

A few scant hours later, I stood in front of the hotel with some other runners in the predawn darkness, waiting for transport to the starting line at the University of Cape Town. The others were visiting Germans. One, in fact, was here on his honeymoon. I wondered whether he had even bothered to tell his bride that he was racing, or whether he was hoping to finish before she awoke. As the van sped along the highway, we talked about our hopes for the race and offered each other energy bars.

The van dropped us off on the main commercial street near to the University, in the suburb of Newlands. I wished the Germans good luck and joined the throng of runners making their way to the starting line. Despite the darkness, it was already quite warm, and I quickly shed my throwaway long-sleeved shirt. I settled into a spot in the crowd behind the starting line, and listened to the last-minute instructions that bellowed from the speakers. The various countries represented were named, to sporadic cheers and applause, and certain notable runners were introduced. The crowd then sang the traditional African song "Shozaloza."

Finally, the announcements were over, and I felt my body tense as I awaited the start, my finger poised on my watch's start button. The gun roared at precisely 6 A.M. I surged forward with the crowd, buoyed by a familiar wave of adrenaline. The asphalt below my feet, smiling faces and cheers of the onlookers, the sight of the runners around me, and even the smells of the race all seemed familiar. The gap in my worldview quickly closed, and Africa, wonderful and exotic, also became, for me, simply another place to run.

As we streamed along the dark city streets, I thought about my race preparation. I had trained for the Two Oceans Marathon as I had trained for the JFK 50 Miler: by including a full marathon in my final long run. This time it was the Virginia Creeper Marathon, a beautiful race in that state's southwest corner which I ran with my friends Dave and Renata. It was my ninty-sixth marathon.

The Two Oceans Marathon has a unique system for awarding finishers' medals. Rather than dividing the field into elite runners and everyone else, the organizers reward different levels of achievement. Runners breaking the 4-hour barrier in the race earn a silver medal, and those breaking 6 hours earn a bronze. Previously, the race had a 6 hour time limit, but now runners who beat 7 hours earn a blue medal. However, many veteran marathoners still consider 6 hours to be the "official" time limit. Factoring in my recent training, jetlag, and the great unknown of the two ascents, I pegged myself as coming in somewhere between 5:15 and 5:30, placing me solidly in the bronze group. In those first few minutes of the race, I calculated the pace necessary to hit my goal, and settled back into an easy stride.

As the sun broke the darkness, I looked at the runners around me. Although they looked like any race field I would find back in the United States, I quickly noticed one key difference: their conversations. Many spoke in the native tongues of South Africa, and even when their conversation dropped into English, the clipped cadences of Afrikaans or Zulu remained. Despite this language barrier, I still felt our bonds as runners, and enjoyed the voices around me.

Passing the first refreshment station, I realized another novelty of the race: there were no rows of cups, as are found in most other races I've run in the United States and abroad. In Cape Town, volunteers handed out water and sports drink in sealed plastic pouches. I ripped a hole in the pouch with my teeth and squirted the water into my mouth.

Newlands gave way to Kenilworth, which became Plumstead, and the city melted into open spaces and small towns. I spotted the pacer for the 6-hour finishers' group, and I reasoned that as long as I keep that group behind me, I would be certain to have a bronze finisher's medal. I passed them and didn't look back.

Being new to the race, I asked several other runners about the course as we ran, and was introduced to another unusual feature of the course: all runners who persevere through ten editions of the race are awarded a permanent blue number to mark their achievement. For me, this meant that veteran ultramarathoners were easier to locate and probe for words of wisdom. They seemed more than willing to oblige.

We entered the town of Lakeside, and then Muizenberg, which gave us our first views of water. This is False Bay, and beyond it the Indian Ocean, the first of the two oceans for which the race is named. The road fell before us as we passed old stone homes in St. James and Kalk Bay, and then, as we entered Fish Hoek and turned inland, we were greeted by a young couple painted entirely in green, cheering us as we streamed past. The views were beautiful and there was still plenty of energy in my legs. These were the good miles.

As I felt energy surge through me, I spied a runner up ahead holding a banner aloft. I wondered if he could possibly be the pacer for sub-5-hour group. No, it couldn't be. But it was. I caught them and stuck to them like glue. As we ran, I asked the pacer about the South African racing circuit. Although the Two Oceans seemed to be a challenging course, he told me that many runners use it as preparation for the Comrades Ultramarathon that follows several months later in mid-June.

Wow. Using a brutal 56-kilometer race as a training run for a more difficult race? There were definitely some tough runners out here.

We ran through Sun Valley, and entered the town of Noordhoek, at kilometer 28, the halfway point of the race. Craft shops and restaurants lined the road, eventually giving way to trees and parkland. Chappies lay just ahead. Our pacer announced that it was time to go to work.

The Chapman's Peak Drive, the race route, was opened to the public in 1922. A popular tourist and sporting destination, it actually consists of two peaks: "Little Chappies," at the 30 kilometer mark of the race, followed by "Big Chappies" 4 kilometers later.

Stands of trees thinned and then disappeared altogether, and the grass melted away as we began our first ascent. The sun was shining brightly now, but I felt comfortable and strong as we followed the road upward. The incline actually felt like a nice change from the earlier flats, and I was surprised at how good I felt. Soon the pace group crested the first summit, and we eased into a short easy stretch of road before the next peak. Talking to the pacer, I learned that the difficulty with Chappies is often not the actual climb, but rather the quick descent that follows, which can wreak havoc with the quads. But other than keeping proper form and trying not to go too fast, there wouldn't be much I could do about that. After all, I never expected to get through this race without some pain.

My thoughts were interrupted by the pacer's announcement that we would resume climbing around the next curve. Feeling confident after conquering Little Chappies, I surged forward ahead of the pack, and after rounding the corner, was able to see the road ahead as it wound its way to the top of Big Chappies. The ascent was over 2½ kilometers, but the views were even more spectacular than they had been from the van window a few days earlier.

Finally, I was at the top of Chappies. Fear that had been gnawing at me since signing up for the race melted away. The climb of Constantia Nek still loomed ahead, but with 17 kilometers left to go, things were looking very, very good. My legs swallowed the descent without a problem, and I said a silent farewell to Chappies as we entered Hout Bay.

Hout Bay was the site of a battle between the Dutch settlers and a British naval force in September, 1795. The Dutch were victorious in a battle that resulted in little loss of life, and cannons used in that victory still guard the town to this day. The proud residents of "the Republic of Hout Bay" have maintained a tradition of firing a cannon as the lead runners enter the town, though I was too far back of the lead pack at that point to hear anything other than the sound of thousands of feet slapping the asphalt. But the spectators and refreshments along the streets of Hout Bay were still a welcome sight.

At about this time fatigue began to seep into my legs, and my earlier soaring confidence started to leak out. I realized that I would probably not be able to maintain the sub-5-hour pace, but I resolved to stay with the group to the 42.1 kilometer mark. I would not have a sub-5-hour finish this day, but making it to the regulation marathon distance with this pack would be my moral victory.

Time ebbed past as I continued to press forward, clinging to the pace group. Finally, I saw an inflated archway spanning the road up ahead—it was the 42.1 kilometer mark. I had earned my victory in the race-within-a-race. As I crossed the timing mat set up near the distance marker, I fought the urge to consider the race finished. The visual cues all said that I'd completed a marathon, and my body certainly felt like it had finished a marathon. Like trained dogs sensing when it is time to go home, my legs were sure that it was time to downshift into cool down mode. Not yet, I told them. There was one last big challenge immediately ahead: Constantia Nek.

With a climb of 215 meters, Constantia Nek is actually the biggest hill on the course, higher even than Big Chappies. But it's also a completely different hill than Chappies. Gone were the cliffs and commanding bayside views; here, the roadside was thick with trees and dotted with residences. The race organizers, knowing that this was where the most suffering would occur, squeezed refreshment stations closer together here, and spectators lined the roads in groups to cheer us on.

At first, the climb didn't seem bad at all. But just as I started to relax, the road suddenly soared up toward the treetops. I had earlier resolved to run the ascents, but this stretch of road made me break that promise, and I briefly joined those who were walking the worst parts of the climb. The strained faces of the runners—runners in name only at this point—mirrored my own determination. Finally, I could see the top of the hill just ahead, and, like a swimmer reaching for poolside, I surged forward with one last push and crested the summit. Constantia Nek was history. Only 10 kilometers left to go.

With all of the fearsome hills finally behind me, I settled into the final task of finishing the race. I shortened my stride and searched for my last reserves of energy as I ran the rolling hills of Rhodes Drive down to the open, sun-drenched avenues of Kirstenbosch, where the glorious Gardens are found. There was now less than 6 kilometers to go. The bright sunlight pulled sweat from our bodies, but I saw no quitters around me. Up ahead was the sweeping turn known as "Harry's Corner," named for a course marshal who manned that corner for years until his death.

The crowd of spectators thickened as we entered Rondebosch, and with it, the university and its football field, where the finish line waited. Mustering the last of my strength, I sprinted to meet it. My final time was 5 hours 15 minutes, the exact time that I had originally hoped for.

As I slowly moved through the crowd, my newly awarded bronze medal hanging around my neck, someone pressed an application for the New York City Marathon into my hand. I continued moving, grabbing fluids and a goody bag, and made my way to the steps leading out of the university and down to the main thoroughfare, to catch a city bus back to Greenmarket Square. As I sat on the bus, an anomalous figure among the Sunday riders, I considered the race application in my hand. I had traveled so far, had experienced so much, but this piece of paper in my hand shrunk all that, shrunk the world. It was as if I had journeyed to the farthest reaches of the North Pole, beyond the edge of civilization, only to find a note from my family waiting for me. And then I realized what I'd always suspected was true: the world is indeed a matrix of running paths, all connected together, stretching from Haile Gebrselassie's flying feet to Chapman's Peak and over to Central Park in Manhattan. In a few short hours I would board a jet back to the States, but standing there with that paper in my hand, I knew that I was already home.

Only one final thing to resolve, though: did this race belong on my list or not? It was billed as a marathon, so that would seem to settle the issue. But it was not the standard marathon distance; it was about 9 miles longer, so it was an ultramarathon. As much as I would have like to have counted this race toward my 100, I knew that could not be allowed. I had now officially run ninety-six marathons and *two* ultramarathons. End of discussion.

Running Tip #17

Trail Running

- *Keep your weight over your feet and shorten your stride.* This will allow you to shift your weight quickly if your footing is unstable.

- *Don't zone out.* Running a trail requires focus and concentration, since a sudden misstep can lead to a debilitating injury. But focus isn't fear. Look at trails as puzzles to be solved.

- *Get the right gear.* Trail-running shoes are best because of their thicker outsoles and better traction. Bring a mini first-aid kit and water; there are no fountains in the woods.

- *Be safe.* Trails, even urban ones, are much more isolated than roads. Use common sense: don't run with an mp3 player or in the dark, since you need to be aware of what's around you, and run with a friend if possible.

Almost There: Marathon Number 99, Wilmington, Delaware

On the morning of May 15, 2005, Dave and I stood in front of Frawley Stadium in Wilmington, Delaware. We were among a small group of people shaking their legs nervously, pacing back and forth, and tying and retying their shoes. I was at another starting line, waiting for the signal that would launch us forward.

We were lucky to be there. Earlier in the morning Dave and I had checked out of our nearby hotel and got in our car for the short drive over to the start. It was about a mile away, a distance that we could easily have jogged or walked, which is exactly what we should have done. Driving on unfamiliar roads, though, we somehow wound up on the entrance ramp to I-95, the major interstate that runs through Wilmington. Peering out the window, I could see people gathering at the starting line as it receded into the distance at 55 miles per hour. I was annoyed, but it wasn't a major problem; we would just get off and turn around.

Except that we couldn't. After getting off the highway at the very next exit, we realized that we weren't near an entrance onto the highway heading back. We had to try our luck on local roads, and ended up having to stop off at a gas station to ask for directions. With scant minutes to spare before the start, I couldn't believe what a mess we had made of things. There was silence in the car as we made our way back, and only after we parked with enough time to walk to the start did we finally relax. Even after all these years of racing, I couldn't take anything for granted.

The prerace dinner had not gone smoothly either. The brochure promised pasta with vegetables and chicken for all runners who attended, which sounded great, but whoever had arranged the meal clearly did not understand the crowd that would be showing up to be fed. A pasta station was set up with chefs cooking up meals to order; a nice touch, but not a very efficient way to feed hundreds of people. As time slipped by, runners grumbled on line and started to fill up on bread and dessert. I managed to finally get some pasta, but it was an unwelcome detour from my prerace regimen.

Despite the setbacks, I felt relaxed at the starting line. I was finally right where I was meant to be, feeling good and loose. It was a warm day, but not a bad one for racing. Clouds lingered from the rain that had blown through overnight, and a light breeze stirred the air. The deputy mayor made a few brief remarks, and a young lady sang "The Star Spangled Banner." And then we were off.

The course was mostly flat, consisting of four loops along the waterfront, the stadium, and an outlet shopping mall. I set out at a comfortable pace, sticking with Dave for a time until he dropped back. I set off on my own, lost in thought, reminiscing about my eighteen years of marathoning. I thought about the ambulances I'd seen out on various racecourses. There is a dark emptiness that marathoners feel anytime they see or hear an ambulance, and I've seen too many of those over the years. I've also seen runners throwing up, lying flat on their backs on the asphalt, and sitting dejectedly on curbs. One friend running the Marine Corps Marathon on an unseasonably hot day made it as far as mile 23 before she collapsed, only to awaken in a medical tent, buried under bags of ice. She recovered fully, but it was a very close call. I thought about how lucky I've been over the years to never have needed those ambulances, and to have escaped major injury. Despite the great demands I had put on my body, it had never broken, and had never given up completely.

I hadn't bothered to look at my watch as I crossed the first two mile markers, which was unusual for me. I suddenly wondered if I could manage to avoid looking at my watch for the entire race. Could I stand not counting the seconds and minutes as they passed? I wanted to be able to do that, to run the race by feel alone, as an experiment in "Zen running." As I finished the first lap, though, I passed beneath the official timing clock, and couldn't help glancing up. Just that quickly, my little experiment was over.

And then came the difficult miles, which every marathoner knows are out there somewhere on the course, the miles that test our will. Four laps in Wilmington were like the four laps of a mile on the track: the first lap is filled with energy and hopefulness; the second lap is for settling into a strong pace and holding it; the third lap is where the pain and doubt set in, when so much running is behind you, but where the finish line is still so far away; and the fourth lap is for just hanging on, where you try to not spoil all the hard work that preceded it.

I ran the race like I was running a hard mile, feeling all the ups and downs of my journey. Each lap on the course had an out-and-back portion, meaning that I was able to see many of the runners in front and behind me. I saw Dave on each lap, as well as the lead runners, striding easily like gazelles. There was a man running in pink tutu; Dave later accused him of lacking the proper respect for the race. I didn't mind—at least it was a distraction.

Finally, I set out on the fourth and final lap. I came upon an older man standing by himself on a street corner, wearing a shirt and tie. He was handing out free bottles of water, and near as I could tell, was not a race volunteer, but just a local resident who thought we needed and deserved to have some support. I took a bottle and thanked him, and then doused myself, feeling the coolness bring strength back to my tired muscles, even if only for a few moments.

Four laps provided enough time for the runners and the race volunteers to come to know each other, even if only in passing. As I passed one volunteer at mile 24, I told him that I hoped he wouldn't take it the wrong way if I said that I was happy not to have to see him again. He laughed and told me to get going.

And then, finally, the finish line was just ahead. As I crossed the line, the official clock overhead read 3:35:07. I had run my 99th marathon 10 minutes and 23 seconds faster than I had run my first one. The Me-That-Is had beaten the Me-That-Was. Someday, I knew, I would no longer be able to beat the Me-That-Was. But that day had not yet come, not in Wilmington.

And now, after all these years and all these miles, there was just one more marathon to go.

Running Tip #18

Eat to Run, Eat to Live

- *Eat a balanced diet:* 65 percent complex carbohydrates, 25 percent lean protein, 10 percent fat, preferably unsaturated vegetable fat, like olive oil.
- *Avoid processed foods and fried foods, and limit your intake of sweets.*
- *Aim to eat a good variety, especially fruits and vegetables.* The brightest and most colorful pack the biggest punch.
- *Graze.* Have something every two hours or so to avoid hunger and binging.
- *Take a daily multivitamin.* How many of us really have a perfect diet? No one I know. So cover your bases.
- *Don't skip breakfast.* You might lose more fat that way, but your workouts will suffer. With your tank full, you'll train better, race better, and lose excess pounds anyway.
- *Watch your portion size.* You should be able to fit most meals in the palm of your hand.
- *Read food labels.* You might be surprised at what's in there. Generally, if the list of ingredients is more than four or so lines long, it's not really food anymore.
- *Low-fat desserts aren't necessarily low-calorie!* These products often still have lots of sugar, so eat sparingly.

Marathon Number 100!

Back in 1987, my supply of running gear consisted of a simple pair of running shoes, a cotton T-shirt, and gym shorts. Nearly two decades down the road, my closet looked much different. On the floor were several pairs of running shoes, costing over $100 each, that were ultra-light and packed with all manner of hi-tech wizardry. On an overhead shelf were neatly folded shirts made of space age breathable fabrics, sporting evocative brand names like Gore-Tex, Dri-FIT, and CoolMax. On a rack hung several breathable, wind and water resistant jackets, and on another shelf sat my wrap-around sunglasses that block out UV rays and random ambient light.

Strapped to my wrist was a watch that could count and store up to 100 interval splits, although it was considered a dinosaur because it couldn't also measure my heart rate, or triangulate with orbiting satellites to record my route and speed. Of course, if I wanted to measure my route, there were now several Web sites that allowed me to precisely calculate the distance I ran, indicating elevation changes as well. In a drawer sat my mp3 digital player, although I usually didn't bring that along on my runs, since I feared getting too dependent on it.

My kitchen had undergone some changes as well. Although I still stocked whole-grain cereals, lean meat, fish, low-fat dairy, and unprocessed fruits and vegetables, I also now used engineered food, such as energy bars, sports drinks, and gels.

Change had also come to the races I ran. Online registration had largely replaced the ritual of mailing in a check and a race application, and the electronic timing chip is now used not only in major marathons, but in races of all distances. And the races themselves have grown larger than I ever thought possible. A field of 20,000 marathoners is now common, and the largest races are nearly double that size.

None of these changes had come about overnight, even if it felt that way to me. But as much as both my own life and the world of marathoning had changed over the years, one thing was constant: more than anything else, I just wanted to run.

And so I had. Now, impossibly, improbably, Dave and I were both about to take our final steps toward achieving our long-held dream. One hundred marathons. Over the years, I kept running, trying not to focus too much on that distant goal. So much could have gone wrong, but now it was really about to happen. I suddenly felt more nervous about it than ever. Which race should it be?

I pored over marathon listings, compared different race courses, and contemplated logistics. Finally, Dave and I made our choice. After coming so far, we wouldn't cut any corners now; we were going to run one of the most grueling races in North America: Grandfather Mountain. Set in the Blue Ridge Mountains in the town of Boone, North Carolina, it represented everything I loved about the marathon. It was beautiful, but after starting at 3,333 feet, it climbed almost 1,000 feet to the peak for which it's named. But it wasn't the net elevation gain that made this race so ominous; there were also numerous drops and climbs along the way. The course elevation profile posted on the race Web site looked like a shark's toothy grin. And to top it all off, the final 4 miles to the finish line were almost entirely uphill.

It was a race that was guaranteed to plumb every runner's well of courage and resolve. But to those who made it to the top came bragging rights, and the sense of accomplishment that only comes from facing a dragon and staring it down. I had learned the hard way over the years never to take a marathon for granted; there were simply too many things that could go wrong. But with Grandfather Mountain, even careful preparation might not be enough. If I could conquer this course, I would have truly earned my record.

Dave agreed that this would be a fitting capstone to our 100-marathon quest. Our friend Renata and another marathoner, Greg, committed to joining Dave and me for our milestone adventure.

Our first challenge would be simply getting there. We opted to make the seven-hour drive the day before the race. When we finally arrived at our hotel on the outskirts of town, we dragged our stiff and sore bodies out of our car and acknowledged to each other with silent looks that this was a less-than-ideal way to prepare for a race.

We were quickly distracted by the strange, mournful sound of a hotel guest practicing her bagpipes in the parking lot. It turned out that the Scottish Highland Games were also being held that weekend on Grandfather Mountain. They were the second largest such games in the world, and the marathon was actually being run in cooperation with them; runners who survived the climb would finish with a victory lap around the competition field, and were welcome to stay afterward and watch the rest of the day's events. This was clearly going to be a race to remember, if only I could make it to the finish.

We went to Appalachian State University to pick up our race numbers and official T-shirts, and to scout out the start of the race, which would be on the university's track at Kidd Brewer Stadium. We then spent the rest of the day wandering around downtown.

Boone was clearly a college town, with cafés and coffee shops lining the main street. It had apparently experienced some recent growth, but it still managed to retain much of an older, enduring charm. I wandered into a small barber shop for a haircut. This had become a little tradition of mine; I had originally started getting haircuts on race weekend simply to kill time and get a chore done, but I also got a little psychological boost from the grooming, since a haircut left me feeling lighter, leaner and faster. I also found that getting a haircut is also a great way to get to know a town if you can get the barber talking. The barber shop in Boone proved especially friendly, and I soon knew not just everything about the town, but all about the barber's own family as well. By the time I stepped back out to the street, I felt that I really knew the place.

On race day, we joined a small but determined group of 400 runners. At the sound of the starting horn, we set off for a single lap around the track, and then exited the stadium for a lap of the parking lot. In any other race, I would have been antsy to hit the roads and get to the meat of the race, but here I knew what lay ahead, and I wasn't in any such hurry.

Finally, we left the university grounds. We cruised past a row of fast-food joints and restaurants and ran toward the town of Blowing Rock. From there we turned onto the scenic Blue Ridge Parkway, and began the climb toward Grandfather Mountain. Here, hills were measured in miles, not feet or yards, and the lush green beauty of our surroundings failed to completely distract any of us from the difficulty of our climbing. I found myself pushing off from my backside with each step, as if I were ascending a ladder instead of running a race.

As I pushed on, I fell into conversation with several other runners. There were clearly a lot of race veterans in this crowd. These runners seemed to love the race not despite the hills, but because of them. With each conquered hill, I began to understand why. Year after year, these runners hurl themselves against the mountain, and are enriched by the experience. The hills stripped away all other concerns, and left us focused on achieving one simple goal: making it to the top. In the process, it would reveal our worst or best selves.

The hills came and went with jarring regularity, until I became accustomed to their rhythm, as if I were standing offshore and weathering a steady surge of waves. Suddenly, the road turned into a gravel and dirt path that rose before me like a wall. It looked so utterly preposterous that I laughed out loud, but I had no choice but to grit my teeth, churn my arms, and attack. With each step I became more determined not to stop running. It was as if eighteen years of marathoning were distilled into this one moment, and I needed to prove that my will was stronger than this latest obstacle. I had decided that if I could make it to the top of that hill, I would finish the race and could claim ownership of my dream, but if I failed, it was all a hoax. It would all come down to this.

Having raised the stakes to that level, I couldn't let myself fail. I sucked in great gulps of air and drove my legs and arms. My eyes blurred with effort; I felt like I was climbing this hill more than running it. A voice in the back of my mind told me that it would be okay to stop, but I pushed that aside. The crest of the hill was now just a few steep yards ahead. No matter how much it hurt, I couldn't stop now. After eighteen years of running, I could not let it end here. Push, I told myself. Push!

And then I had done it; I was king of the hill. I still had miles left to go, but I knew the race was effectively over. Whatever lay ahead, it would not, could not, defeat me.

Still, it could hurt. The final few miles were mostly uphill as promised. The very last stretch passed the aid tent where food and drink were available for finishers—a cruel sight for runners who hadn't yet crossed the finish line. The road rose up toward the make-shift arena; it was an incline that earlier would have worried me, but I had come too far now and conquered too much already. I crested Grandfather Mountain, and entered McRae Meadows. Passing through the crowd, I entered the arena for my victory lap on the dirt track, buoyed by the applause and cheers of the spectators. I pulled my form together and asked my tired, sore legs for just one more effort, a burst of speed to give the spectators something to cheer about. Just a few more minutes of agony, and it would all be over. My legs agreed, and they propelled me across around the final curve and across the finish line. I checked my watch: 3 hours, 46 minutes, 25 seconds. Eighteen years after my first marathon, I had finally arrived.

One hundred marathons. It was done.

Dave came in a short time later, and I and cheered him as he, too, crossed the finish line. He had reached his 100-marathon milestone as well. We had run some thirty marathons together; a friendship forged on roads and trails, spanning more race miles together than most runners compile in their entire lives. That crazy idea we had concocted years earlier had somehow come true. Now we grinned, shook hands, and hugged.

Now that my race was over, I felt fatigue, but mostly relief and joy. Not just for having survived one of the toughest races in the country, but to have had the right combination of determination and luck to have reached my goal. Dave and I gobbled down some peanut butter sandwiches, grabbed some drinks, and settled into the stands to watch some of the Highland Games as we waited for Renata and Greg to come into view. On the field, athletes were doing something that could only be described as a telephone-pole toss. Just watching them made my back ache, and I realized that in this crowd, running a marathon probably looked like a tame thing to do.

Finally, our little group was reunited, and we made our way to the Scottish Clan reunion area, where booth displays honored different family lines. I didn't expect to see any tables for Clan Horowitz, but Dave found some distant brethren.

On the long ride home, we had plenty of time to consider what we had achieved. In the coming days, I thought about all those race miles, and tried to wrap my head around the immensity of it. I had raced in fourty-six states, thirteen countries, and four continents (not including my ultramarathon in South Africa). I had run up and down mountains, across deserts and lava fields, through forests, vineyards, and cities. I had met many extraordinary people, and witnessed the very best of human nature. I had, I believed, lived life to the fullest.

But did I remember it all? Such a strange question. I certainly remembered each marathon, but did I remember every minute of each one? No, of course not. My 100 marathons had cumulatively taken about 385 hours to run. That's over sixteen days of non-stop, round-the-clock racing. Who can recall every minute of a single hour, let alone sixteen entire days? But still, I was surprised at how few minutes I did recall. I remembered certain moments from each race when I saw something interesting, or when I crossed the finish line, but all the other moments were lost to me.

I have memories, however, that are untethered to any specific race. I experience random flashbacks of running beneath sun-dappled leaves along a tree-lined street, or past a row of shops, and I can't link those memories with any particular race. It's a bit like finding an old photograph wherein you recognize yourself, but not all of the people around you. You knew them once, but no longer. It's an uncomfortable, disconcerting feeling.

Equally disturbing was a realization that I had midway through a recent race. I suddenly knew that I'd soon forget most of what I was seeing around me. I ran past ordinary office buildings and plain houses, thinking, "I'll forget that one, and that one, and that one, too." It was as if I was erasing my life almost as fast as my mind was recording it. Then I realized that this realization applied not just to my racing, but to our lives in general, since most of our day-to-day experience is lost to us as time goes by. Perhaps that's for the best, since our memories would be a chaotic sea of details if our minds didn't filter out unimportant minutiae.

Still, I wouldn't trade a single minute of this racing life, whether I remembered each of them or not. But what could I do for an encore? The answer was as simple as it was predictable: check the calendar and fill out my next race application. There were four states still remaining for me to conquer to be able to claim having run marathons in them all. Then the Canadian provinces—of which I'd already done three—and then the last three of the seven continents I hadn't yet raced on. Then there were dream race destinations, like the Himalayas and the Machu Picchu trail, and beautiful cities around the globe that boasted breathtaking marathons, like Prague, Madrid, Venice, and London. There would never be a shortage of marathons that could quicken my pulse and capture my imagination.

I thought about an advertising campaign put on not long ago by a major running-shoe company. It featured the slogan "There is no finish line." But rather than finding myself inspired, I was demoralized. Without a finish line, I had no sense of accomplishment, no valid way to measure my journey. Without finish lines, my running would consist of endless miles, as devoid of perspective as the emptiness of space, as empty of joy as boundless time. I need finish lines as much as I need the seasons, a calendar, and a watch. But these finish lines are not ends; they are only a brief rest stop before the next race. I had now crossed one hundred of these finish lines, but the journey wasn't over; I'd already begun planning my next 100.

Running Tip #19

The Last Supper

The best race preparation can be undermined by bad eating decisions the night before a race. Don't make that mistake.

- *Eat early.* You don't want to feel bloated at the starting line.
- *Don't over-eat.* Carb-loading doesn't mean carb-gorging. Eat a relatively light meal early, and have a light snack before bedtime.
- *Avoid foods you haven't tried before.* Choose a carb, like pasta, rice, or bread, and a protein, like lean meat, skinless poultry, or low-fat dairy. It doesn't have to be bland, but don't be adventurous.
- *Hydrate!* Avoid alcohol and caffeinated drinks.

Why Run the Marathon? Bell Lap: Running & Remembrance

In middle-distance races held on a track, race officials let the runners know when they're on their final lap by ringing a bell. This is the bell lap, the lap that determines the winner. It's the lap that counts.

I'm now in the bell lap of my story. I have traveled all over the world, running marathons, celebrating life. Along the way, I've pondered why I ran. I reached my goal; and I've told my story, but I still have one last chapter to write; I still need an answer to that question: why run the marathon?

I thought about a recent trip I'd taken back up to Queens, New York, to visit friends and family. That Saturday morning, I set out on a run. It was early, and after stepping out of the apartment where I'd been raised, I began running down the old familiar streets of my youth, past stores where I held after-school jobs, past school yards where I used to spend long summer days playing handball and stickball. I ran past Alley Pond Park, where my friends and I would occasionally do short runs on a bike trail through the woods. Back then, our 3-mile run seemed like a tremendous achievement.

I left the park and headed west on Union Turnpike, a major thoroughfare that ran past the apartment complex where I lived. Every weekday morning from age twelve through eighteen, I would board the Q44 bus on Union

Turnpike for the 6 mile ride to the train station, where I would take the F train to the N train to the uptown 7, exiting at 96th Street for the short walk to my school. It was an hour-and-a-half commute, but that didn't seem unusual to me. Everyone in New York commutes.

As I ran down the avenue, I thought about my father. He used to take the Q44 bus also, getting off earlier to transfer to another bus to nearby Jamaica Avenue and the clothing store where he worked. After I moved to D.C. and became a runner, I ran along this bus route when I was visiting. I'd try to keep pace with each bus as it passed, looking to see if my father was on board, on his way to work. He always stood toward the back of the bus, a figure in a dark raincoat, looking out the window, leaning in to get a better view, looking for me as I was looking for him, waving at me as I waved back.

My father and I, like many fathers and sons, weren't very close, though I think we both wanted to be. We had difficulty talking with one another, of finding common ground. This chasm grew when I went to college and entered a world that he had no experience with. It would be many years until I began to understand that he showed more character through his daily sacrifice for his family than I would ever learn in school. It is a lesson that I continue to learn. But on those runs back home, I didn't yet understand these things, so the brief morning encounters we had, with me on foot and him peering through the bus window, were one of the few ways we had of connecting.

My parents were actually very proud of my running. Even Dad, who never let on when he approved of anything his children had done, bragged about me to his coworkers, and when I gave him a plaque with mounted photos of me crossing the finish line, he showed it to anyone who would be foolish enough to agree to see it. Dad wasn't an athletic man; in fact, he was often quite overweight. I had the feeling that my running somehow balanced the scales for him, that by producing someone who could accomplish these things, he had shown that it was in him somewhere as well.

Then, in 1988, right after I graduated from law school, I decided that I wanted to go skydiving. It sounded like a fun thing to do. My parents weren't so proud of that decision. They thought me foolish for wanting to throw myself out of a plane after all the hard work I put in to getting through law school. It was all fine and good to run marathons—even if I didn't win any of them, as my dad once pointed out—but at least that was safe. You get tired, you stop. Easy. But what sane person jumps out of a plane?

We never agreed on it, but one sunny day, I did it anyway. It was a static line jump, like in those old World War II movies where paratroopers dove out the door and their chutes opened automatically, except in my case there was no diving. Each of us crawled out to the edge and then slid out the door, hanging onto the strut of the overhead wing, waiting for the signal to let go from the jumpmaster, who sat just inside the door. I was third of three to go, and after sucking in engine fumes as our plane circled, climbing and dropping, I was more than ready to jump. I crawled out and looked up for the instructor's thumbs-up sign. He gave it, and I let go.

I didn't get a free fall, didn't get to assume the arch position that the instructor had us practice earlier. As it turned out, my chute opened almost immediately after I let go of the plane. But I did get some fine gliding time under the canopy, circling left and right as I tugged on the toggles above me.

I slowly drifted down to the target landing spot on the field. I misjudged my distance from the ground, though, so I landed hard and rolled instead of stepping gracefully back onto the earth. Not perfect, but good. And very fun.

I called my parents afterward. I hadn't told them that this was the day I would be jumping; no point in having them spend the day gazing at the clock, wondering if I'd splattered yet. They were relieved that I got through it okay, and that I had gotten it out of my system. Except that I hadn't. My jump was fun, but a free fall, well, that would be something else altogether. I needed just a few more jumps to graduate to that level. It would be easy.

My parents didn't share my enthusiasm. In fact, Dad started a letter-writing campaign against it. Well, he didn't actually write any letters. Instead, he clipped articles on gruesome skydiving accidents and sent them to me, without even attaching a note. Stories like the one about the skydiver who got tangled up in a plane's fuselage and had to cut himself loose from his chute to save the plane, while dooming himself. I wondered where he found these; I had never seen a single one on my own.

I knew that I'd have to deal with this sooner or later, or one of us would crack. I needed a plan.

Here's what I came up with: while Dad was always overweight, he would occasionally add on an extra twenty pounds or so, which he would drop as soon as his coworkers started teasing him about it. He'd gotten big again recently, and wasn't losing weight, despite the teasing. So I offered Dad a deal: no more skydiving if he lost forty pounds and kept it off. There seemed to be no downside there for me; if he agreed, he would either lose the weight, but probably put it back on later, freeing me from my bond, or he wouldn't lose the weight, and would have forfeited his right to campaign against me, since he knew exactly what he had to do to get me to stop. Brilliant.

Dad agreed to the deal. Then he quickly lost the forty pounds. That surprised me, but I was okay with it, because I knew that the game wasn't over yet. Then something unexpected happened; he seemed pale and tired easily, and Mom said that he was getting night sweats. That wasn't part of my plan.

We talked Dad into seeing his doctor, who took blood samples and ordered some tests. I figured Dad's crash diet had left him with some type of anemia, and the doctor said yes, that there was evidence of anemia, but he also said that there was something more. He wanted to take some tests. So Dad took off a week from work and let the doctor poke and prod and stick him. After all that, the doctor announced that he wanted to do a bone-marrow biopsy.

For me, that was the first sign that something might be seriously wrong.

I went up to New York that weekend, right before the biopsy was scheduled to be performed, to spend time with my parents and with my younger sister, Dori. My older sister, Marlene, was abroad traveling, but we were keeping her updated. While I was home, we just relaxed, and spent time poring through old photographs. We found some of Mom and Dad's wedding shots, and laughed at Dad's terrified expression, looking at us across the decades with great big eyes.

I was back at work on Monday when I got a phone call from a neighbor telling me that my dad was ill, and that I needed to come up immediately. I called my mother to find out exactly what was going on, and she could only say, "He's gone, he's gone." Finally, she told me that Dad had just collapsed and died. I jumped on the next flight to New York.

I sat gazing out the window, tears welling in my eyes, waiting for the flight to be over, but wishing that the plane would never land. An elderly woman sitting beside me started up a conversation. More than a decade later, I still wonder whether she somehow guessed what had happened, and was just trying to distract me.

She asked what I did for a living. I told her that I was an attorney. Looking at my hands, callused from working out in the gym, she said, "there's no shame in being a workman, you know."

"Yes," I said. "I know. But I really am an attorney."

After I arrived in New York, I kept wondering what it was the doctor had been testing for. I finally called and asked. Lymphoma, he said. Cancer. He was sure of it, and only ordered the biopsy to confirm it. Dad would have been dead within two years, he said. He was surprised at my dad's sudden death, but he said that perhaps it was for the best.

My dad dropping dead was for the best. I rolled that one around in my mind for a while. It was hard to accept, but I knew he was probably right.

But here's what I'm not supposed to tell you: a day or two after I had returned home, I took a late-night walk with my mother. She seemed to want to say something, so I asked her what was on her mind. She told me that on the day Dad died, he had been nervous about the biopsy, and had asked her to lie down with him. Mom paused and looked me in the eyes. "You know what I mean? *Lie down.*" The dime dropped, and I got it.

"Afterward," she continued, "he got up and went into the next room and collapsed." She looked me in the eyes, deadly serious. "Do you think I killed him?"

Good god. Can you imagine? Bad enough to have to think about my parents having sex, but now I had to imagine Mom killing Dad in the sack. *Well,* I thought, *maybe she did. Good for him. Good for her. Good for the both of them! What a great way that would be to go: spend a week at home, have your son come in for a visit, make love to your wife, then go into the next room and check out. That's a pretty sweet deal.*

Of course, I didn't say any of this to my mom. I told her, "Of course not. When it's your time, it's your time, and nothing you did with him could have changed that."

Which might be true. Or perhaps not.

Meanwhile, I was comforted, too, by the realization that my parents had always wanted it to be this way. Not at that exact moment or in that way, but in the scheme of things. Children bury parents; that's how it was supposed to be. Any time we heard about a child dying first, the expression on my parents' faces betrayed pain for the grieving parents that they didn't even know. Looking back, I realized that my parents had, knowingly or not, prepared me for this moment all my life.

I had it in my mind that burying my dad was a very personal thing, and I didn't want a stranger to do it. In Jewish funerals, the immediate family and closest friends each toss a shovelful of dirt on the coffin after it's been lowered down into the earth. After that, workers generally come over and shovel the bulk of the dirt into the grave. It seemed too impersonal to me. Burying my father was my last act of devotion to him, and I wanted to do it myself. My mother and sisters understood, and gave their consent. I then asked my family rabbi if it would be allowed. He warned me that it would be hard work. I smiled, and explained to him that I was in pretty good shape.

And that's how it went. For years afterward, when I ran down Union Turnpike, I couldn't help but glance up at each passing bus, looking to see if my father was on board. I know it makes no sense, but part of me imagined that it would still be possible to see him standing there, waving at me, if only I could run fast enough and catch the right bus. My running would bring him back to me.

I think now about all the other places that I had run over the seasons and the years, the people I met, the person I was, and the person I had become. Running seems to be the thread that connects it all, a line to all that was and all that is; a strip of asphalt thousands of miles long, on which I'd run all the workouts and races of my life.

I wonder what the Runner-That-I-Was would think about the Runner-That-I-Am, and I imagine that if I run really fast, I would be able to fold the years and catch sight of the Me-That-Was. We'd lock eyes in passing, and he'd nod slightly and tip his hand, the runner's greeting that says, "I know you; you are one of us."

My mind floods with the memories of my running in D.C. I recall crossing Key Bridge during a driving rainstorm, and the sweltering heat of the 14th Street Bridge in late summer. I recall the reflection of myself on an office building's gleaming window during a 10K race, and the potholes I've scrambled over, and occasionally stepped into.

I think again about the marathon, and again about the question why. I've lived with the marathon for nearly two decades; it has become a part of my being, my personal culture. It is no longer just something I do; it is a reflection of who I am. The great Czech Olympic champion Emil Zátopek said that if you want to win something, run 100 meters,

Why Run the Marathon? Bell Lap: Running & Remembrance

but if you want to experience something, run a marathon. I've wanted the experience, and I've discovered that each marathon is a life-journey all its own, filled with expectation, disappointment, realization, and, sometimes, triumph. It has become the measure and mirror of my life.

I think again about Burt, my personal training client who passed away. I think about how the muscles we fought so hard to strengthen have now melted from his bones, and that I may be the only one who knows how hard he struggled to improve himself. But I know that Burt labored not just to gain strength and fitness; what Burt gained in the gym was a sense of purpose. His struggles were a demonstration of his character and his faith in the wonder of life. I think, too, about my two team members in Rome, and how we talked about the meaning of the marathon, of the arbitrariness of the number 26.2, of the relative insignificance of finishing times.

Finally, I had my answer. I knew why it was important to run the marathon. The race distance matters, but only because it takes 26.2 miles to strip away the falsehoods and comfortable compromises of daily life. My finishing times matter also, but only as a reflection of my effort. I know that I will eventually lose my speed, and that someday I will get old and die. But during the time I am here, I will find a deeper satisfaction and meaning to my daily routine; I will find a way to connect to the animal that I am, and to make a statement about what kind of person I am, and what I stand for. It doesn't really matter that I will slow and weaken. There is a kind of glory to be found here, a glory earned through sweat and effort, from a stubborn refusal to give less than your best. It is the reward that dwarfs all the medals tucked away in my drawer. It is why I run the marathon.

Here's a story: during the 1968 Olympic Games in Mexico City, the winner of the marathon had already crossed the finish line over an hour earlier when John Stephen Akhwari of Tanzania entered the stadium. Akhwari was limping, and his leg was wrapped in a bloody bandage. Akhwari slowly made his way around the track to the finish line, as the few spectators who remained in the stands applauded his efforts. Afterward, a reporter asked Akhwari why he hadn't just dropped out of the race, since he clearly had no chance of winning. Akhwari paused, and then said, "My country did not send me to Mexico City to start the race. They sent me to finish." It was the greatest last-place finish ever, and perhaps the most succinct expression I'd ever heard of the marathon spirit.

Everyone needs a place to make their stand, to declare their character through their actions, to say "this is who I am and what I believe." For me, that statement begins with a race application and a pair of running shoes. We marathoners are the people who suffer and persevere. That is who we are.

As I write these words, I look over at Stephanie. Soon after we married, we talked about whether we wanted a child. We were both accustomed to an adventurous lifestyle, and we were reluctant and even scared to take on the burden of parenthood. Even if we wanted one, we knew that the odds were against us. We were both forty, which we knew was a problem. Friends our age had gone to extraordinary lengths to conceive, using fertility drugs and in vitro fertilization. We fully expected that would be our lot as well, much as we hoped to avoid it.

We finally decided to try to start a family. Actually, it would be more accurate to say that we decided that we didn't want to *not* have one, which was what we thought would be the result if we put off making a decision any longer. Since we were sure that we would have difficulty getting pregnant anyway, we made an appointment with a clinic. Stephanie showed up for her appointment on time. She'd missed her last period, but she wasn't concerned. These things happen occasionally. The doctor did a few preliminary tests, and then came back with surprising news: we didn't need his services after all. Stephanie was already pregnant.

We were dumbstruck. As Stephanie's belly swelled, the reality of our situation slowly sunk in. In time, we found out that we were going to have a boy, and we began the ritualistic collecting-of-things that all expecting parents go through. I trusted her to decide what we needed; I hadn't even heard of many of the things that she told me were essential, and even holding them in my hands left me with little clear idea of what to do with them.

The one thing I did take responsibility for, though, was the choosing of the jogging stroller. After extensive research, I bought a model that just screamed speed. It looked like it was setting a PR even when it was standing still. I felt ready for our son.

As we got closer to our due date, I thought more about what kind of father I wanted to be, and I began to feel hopelessly ill prepared. How had my father handled it, and his father before him? I hoped that my instincts and basic common sense would carry me through. And I also counted on close supervision by Stephanie.

One thing I did feel confident about, though, was my determination to be a running father. If children really do learn best by example, then my little boy would learn that it's perfectly natural to run on a nice day, and to enter a marathon and finish it. He would watch his old man compete, and see that hundreds and thousands of other dads and moms did the same thing. He would grow up thinking that there was nothing extraordinary or unusual about this, and that he could do it, too, if he wished. He could do anything he wanted, if he did the work.

As I glance over at Stephanie's belly now, I think of the lessons I learned from my father, and I think of how I will some day be regarded by my own son when I'm gone. I hope that he'll recall the passion with which I pursued my dreams, and understand that in my running, I was trying to explain to him my understanding of life, and how to live it. This is the gift I wish to give to my son.

My 100th marathon has now come and gone, less a finish line itself than a marker on a path. More are planned, and after that, more will hopefully follow, stretching into the distance like light posts on an endless highway. As each one comes into view, I will greet it and test myself against it, pushing muscle and sinew against time and distance. If ever I should forget who I am, and what I believe, I only need to run that path, and in my running, I will find my way back to myself, and discover once again who I am.

Epilogue: Bumps in the Endless Road

In November 2004, a story was reported in the back pages of *The New York Times* that was of great interest to me.[8] Dr. Dennis M. Bramble of the University of Utah and Dr. Daniel E. Lieberman of Harvard had published a paper hypothesizing that ancient humans were physiologically predisposed to be long-distance runners.

The scientists had begun by analyzing the evolution of our physique. As early as two million years ago, humans developed an upright posture, long legs, shorter arms and a narrower ribcage and pelvis. We also lost our fur, which allowed us to develop sweat glands and prevent overheating during intense exertion. We developed a ligament network to keep our heads steady while running, and a muscle and tendon network along the back of our legs, including an Achilles tendon, to store and release great amounts of energy—enough to propel our bodies forward quickly with power. And then there's our highly-developed backside, which stabilizes our midsection during running.

---

8 "Even Couch Potatoes May Have Been Born to Run," by John Noble Wilford, *New York Times*, November 17, 2004.

All of these traits are conducive not just to walking, but to long distance running, and apes don't share any of them. Bramble and Lieberman speculated that running would have increased the early humans' chances of survival, as they could cover large areas of African grassland in pursuit of food.

Apparently, then, we are all born to run.

Of course, I knew that already. I was once told that there's a German word, *tatesfruedig,* which roughly means the joy of doing that which you can do well. A cheetah loves to sprint because it is built to sprint, and a monkey loves to climb because it is built to climb. My running wasn't an aberration; it was an expression of my genetic heritage. It was something I was born to do.

So I kept on running. I ran marathons in Montana, Alaska, and North Dakota. In late September, with the birth of my son just days away, I returned to the Marine Corps Marathon yet again. And then, on November 12, 2005, I experienced something more miraculous than a marathon finish line: the birth of Alex Michael, named in honor of my grandfather and Stephanie's dad. I cut his umbilical cord and then later laid my hand across his tiny body. There was no amount of thinking that could compare to the reality I saw before me. It was magical and humbling. I thought about my life, and I felt like I was the luckiest man on earth.

Then things became unhinged. A dear friend of twenty years died of breast cancer. A cousin died from lung cancer. And then hardest of all, I had to watch my mother's health suddenly spiral downward, despite all the treatments recommended by the best doctors we could find. Mom was obese and had diabetes, which I knew was a time bomb waiting to explode, but there was little I could do about it. As a coach and trainer, I felt particularly responsible, but I couldn't force her to save her own life, and after a while, I decided not to spend whatever time we had left together fighting with her over this. But now her problems gained a velocity I never could have imagined: she experienced full renal failure and had to go on dialysis, then she contracted pneumonia twice and a vicious intestinal infection. Fear and various drugs addled her mind, and a foot infection forced her doctors to amputate her leg. The lone bright spot for us was the look on her face when she held tiny Alex in her arms for the first time.

Her health continued to decline. Every time the phone rang, I feared the worst. My sisters and I shuttled Mom between hospitals and nursing homes, and we realized at some point that she would never return to her old apartment. We were still hopeful of her recovery, and had just filed the paperwork to move her into a home that could properly care for her. My sister Marlene was visiting us in D.C. with her two children when we got the phone call from New York. Mom's blood pressure had suddenly plummeted, and she had needed to be resuscitated twice. She now had a tube snaking down her throat, delivering oxygen, and her heart was beating only because she was being fed drugs intravenously. Her doctors wanted to know if we wanted to give them the order to stop resuscitating her. They wanted to know if we were ready to let her die.

Marlene had been on a grand tour of Europe and Asia when Dad fell ill. When she called us from Istanbul, we told her not to worry, but that she should sit still for a while and keep in touch. There was no need to panic, after all. Everything would be okay. And then Dad suddenly died, as you know. Marlene immediately got on a plane heading home, and spent that twelve-hour flight weeping and growing the guilt she would carry forever for not being home when her daddy passed away.

As I looked at Marlene now, I knew that more than anything else, I didn't want Mom to pass away without Marlene being at her bedside. So the answer was no. We would not give a do-not-resuscitate order. We told the doctors to keep the meds flowing. We were on our way.

When we reached the hospital, Stephanie took Alex and Marlene's children back to Marlene's house, where Marlene's husband Jerry was waiting for them. Marlene and I went up to Mom's room in intensive care. Our sister Dori was already there, with red-rimmed eyes. She had been there for hours.

We went right to Mom's bedside. She looked back at us, wide-eyed, gasping for air as a tube hung from her mouth. Her gaze shifted, and I realized that she was looking back and forth across the room. Back and forth, again and again. I wondered if she knew we were there.

We stepped into the hall to speak with the doctors on call. They told us that the only thing keeping Mom alive was the medication they were pumping into her veins to maintain her blood pressure and heartbeat. Mom's body had already begun to shut down; the flow of blood to her remaining leg had virtually stopped. After absorbing this information, we returned to her room. I pulled back the blanket and looked at her right leg. Her foot was already turning black.

My sisters sobbed while they held Mom's hands and stroked her head. I stood at the bedside, waiting. Finally, we looked at each other, and started talking about what needed to be done.

How do you go about stating the obvious when no one wants to hear it? I was a lawyer, so I approached it in a lawyerlike way: I made the case. Mom could not live on her own without these extreme lifesaving measures, and what she had now was not living. Even if she were to somehow revive and not need life support, her remaining leg was rapidly dying, and would need to be removed. Would she be able to survive another amputation? We doubted it.

When we were finished reviewing the situation, we just stood there, not wanting to say what needed to be said. It seemed like we had been led into a Faustian bargain; in exchange for being allowed to be at her mother's bedside at her passing, we had to give the order to let her die. It was an awful responsibility, but as we looked at Mom, the reality sunk in. We realized that we really had no choice at all. It had already happened. We were there to just hold her hand and observe the passage.

We went back out in the hall and summoned the doctors. They told us that if we discontinued the medications, her heart rate would immediately begin to drop. She would probably only start to feel lightheaded, and then gently slip away. After all the months of physical and mental agony she had endured, it seemed only fair that she was at least given a peaceful end.

We had the meds cut off, and my sisters and I stood around her bedside, stroking her face and saying "I love you." I leaned in close to her cheek, kissed her, and whispered, "Be at peace," and then I glanced at the monitor and watched the drop in her heart rate. It fell slowly but steadily, from 119, to 107, to 98. My sisters cried more intensely, and held her hands tightly. Mom still looked up at us wide eyed.

84. 77. 65.

Her cheek felt cold to me, but as soft as it was when I stroked it as a boy. When I was very little I once told her that when she got old, I would get her a facelift. I don't know where I had gotten that idea. I wondered what she thought when I said it.

59. 53. 48. 42.

Her eyes seemed to lose their vitality. I wanted the moment to be over, and I wanted it to never end. I wondered what she was thinking.

36. 28. 19. 12.

Stillness.

After my mother died, I felt numb and detached. Even with Stephanie and Alex beside me, I was shaken by the sudden disappearance of so many people from my life. I didn't know what to do to make it all seem okay, so I relied on the one thing that had always provided me with support when I was troubled: I ran. I raced in Arizona, Florida, Wyoming, and still that was not enough. While Mom was ill, Stephanie and I had made plans to let her mother watch Alex while the two of us went to Mexico for a vacation—and a chance for me to run the Mexico City Marathon. After Mom died, I wasn't sure we should still go, but we decided it would be best for us to stick with our plans. More than anything, we needed some time alone. It was the right choice. We had a wonderful time, even if we missed Alex.

And still I kept running. On October 8, 2006, Dave and I completed the Mt. Rushmore Marathon, crossing the finish line together. We had added the final state to our list, and could now both claim to have run the entire country.

I didn't stop there; I added more and more marathons to my list, running them more frequently than I ever had before. And then I committed the cardinal runner's sin: I ignored pain, thinking it would just go away. It didn't. My body suddenly decided that enough was enough, and grounded me with a series of devastating injuries. Tenderness in my hamstrings, blinding pain in my Achilles tendon, and stabbing pain in my heel. My running came to a screeching halt. I was through.

After a series of X-rays and MRIs, I accepted that I would be off running, and that I would never again run the way I used to. I was allowed to cross-train, and I attacked the bike and weight room with a singled-minded fury, but I missed my running. The weeks passed, and I followed the doctor's orders religiously, but I was still grounded. I kept up a cheerful face for my charity running team and my friends, but I'd never before had to face a setback like this. After all I had just witnessed, I knew that not being able to run was hardly the worst tragedy one could face, but it was still a difficult blow to me. The one crutch that I had consistently relied upon over the years to help me through all my crises was itself in crisis. I felt lost.

In April 2008, I sat in an airport, waiting by a gate for a plane that would take my charity runners and me to Monterey, California for a race along the coast. They would run, but I would not. But I was their coach, and I was committed to helping them achieve their goals. It was all I could do. But in the airport at that moment, I just wanted to sit quietly and read. I didn't want to think about running.

"You ran the Dublin Marathon?"

"Huh?" I said, confused.

"Did you run the Dublin Marathon?" The tall man standing in front of me pointed at my backpack. "It says so on your bag."

"Oh, right. Yeah, I ran that a couple of times. It's a fun race."

"Do you run a lot?"

"Well, not right now, but I used to." And so I told him about my races. Eventually I told him how many I'd run.

"You should write a book."

"Funny you should say that."

"Wait a minute," he said, getting up. "I gotta get someone." He came back with a few people and introduced me. We all sat there and talked running. Races we'd finished, races we'd dreamed of doing, the great moments and the horrible ones. And little by little, I began to feel better.

"Good talking with you," the first man said. "You're an inspiration."

An inspiration. That was funny. They hadn't known how depressed I was just a few minutes earlier. And now like a summer storm, it had blown away. Talking with them, I felt my hope rekindle, and I suddenly knew that these injuries—these terrible but completely common injuries—would pass, and I would solve the puzzle of my body and find a way to run again, to race again. Despite all, the road was not ended and I was not finished. Everything in my life would be all right.

I was still a runner.

By the Numbers

1 Marine Corps Marathon, Washington, D.C., November 8, 1987—3:45:30

2 Marine Corps Marathon, Washington, D.C., November 4, 1990—4:08:00

3 New York City Marathon, November 3, 1991—4:11:12

4 Shamrock Marathon, Virginia Beach, March 20, 1993—3:45:33

5 Pittsburgh Marathon, May 2, 1993—4:25:42

6 Columbia Birthday Marathon, Maryland, September 19, 1993—3:35:00

7 Northern Central Trails Marathon, Maryland, November 27, 1993—4:00:17

8 Boston Marathon, April 18, 1994—3:57:38

9 Vermont Marathon, Burlington, May 29, 1994—3:40:33

10 Grandma's Marathon; Duluth, Minnesota, June 19, 1994—3:47:38

11 Atlantic City Marathon, New Jersey, October 16, 1994—3:39:52

12 New York City Marathon, November 6, 1994—3:42:33

13 Richmond Marathon, Virginia, November 27, 1994—3:35:38

14 Philadelphia Marathon, November 20, 1994—3:43:44

15 Las Vegas Marathon, February 4, 1995—3:58:26

16 LaSalle Chicago Marathon, October 15, 1995—3:21:28

17 Marine Corps Marathon, Washington, D.C., October 22, 1995—4:27:55

18 Schweizer's Delaware Marathon, December 10, 1995—3:34:12

19 Disneyworld Marathon, Orlando, January 7, 1996—3:26:55

20 *Charlotte Observer* Marathon, North Carolina, February 17, 1996—3:28:48

21 Music City Marathon; Nashville, Tennessee, March 16, 1996—3:38:39

22 Cleveland Marathon, May 5, 1996—3:44:39

23 Mayor's Midnight Marathon, Anchorage, June 22, 1996—3:19:41

24 Marine Corps Marathon, Washington, D.C., October 27, 1996—3:37:46

25 Atlanta Marathon, November 28, 1996—3:32:05

26 Kiawah Island Marathon, South Carolina, December 14, 1996—3:23:47

27 25th Olympiad Memorial Marathon, St. Louis, February 23, 1997—3:48:51

28 Ridge Runner Marathon, West Virginia, June 7, 1997—3:40:57

29 San Francisco Marathon, July 13, 1997—3:32:00

30 East Lyme Marathon, Connecticut, September 28, 1997—3:12:57

31 Detroit International Marathon, Michigan, October 19, 1997—3:08:59

32 Vulcan Marathon; Birmingham, Alabama, November 8, 1997—3:31

33 Mardi Gras Marathon; New Orleans, Louisiana, January 17, 1998—3:45:02

34 Lincoln Marathon, Nebraska, May 3, 1998—3:18:05

35 Heroes Marathon; Madison, Wisconsin, May 24, 1998—3:10:09

36 Sunburst Marathon; South Bend, Indiana, June 6, 1998—3:36:50

37 Pikes Peak Marathon, Colorado, August 16, 1998—6:58:00

38 New Hampshire Marathon, October 3, 1998—3:46:00

39 Louisville Marathon, December 5, 1998—3:30:22

40 Houston Marathon, January 19, 1999—3:25:14

41 The Last Marathon, Antarctica, February 13, 1999—5:10:00

42 Los Angeles Marathon, March 14, 1999—3:27:25

43 Boston Marathon, April 19, 1999—3:09:00

44 *Deseret News* Marathon, Utah, July 24, 1999—3:54:00

45 Tupelo Marathon, Mississippi, September 5, 1999—3:32:13 (19/120)

46 Berlin Marathon, September 26, 1999—3:26:17

47 Marine Corps Marathon, Washington D.C., October 24, 1999—3:21:15 (with a borrowed number—sorry, Mr. Race Director!)

48 New York City Marathon, November 7, 1999—3:34:51

49 Seattle Marathon, November 28, 1999—3:32:34

50 Jacksonville Marathon, Florida, December 18, 1999—3:24:15

51 Myrtle Beach Marathon, South Carolina, February 5, 2000—3:15:00

52 B&A Trail Marathon, Maryland, March 12, 2000—3:40:01

53 Boston Marathon, April 17, 2000—3:11:44

54 Portland Marathon, Maine, October 1, 2000—3:22:04

55 Beijing Marathon, October 15, 2000—3:31:01

56 Dublin Marathon, October 30, 2000—3:27:45

57 Honolulu Marathon, December 10, 2000—3:25:37

58 Bermuda Marathon, January 14, 2001—3:23:37 (16/287)

59 Desert Classic Marathon; Phoenix, Arizona, February 18, 2001—3:44:01

60 Rome Marathon, March 25, 2001—3:49:38

61 Boston Marathon, April 16, 2001—3:19:05

62 Vienna City Marathon, May 20, 2001—3:41:37

63 New Mexico Marathon, September 9, 2001—3:33:00

64 Steamtown Marathon; Scranton, Pennsylvania, October 7, 2001—3:20:14

65 Dublin Marathon, October 31, 2001—4:07:00

66 Athens Marathon, Greece, November 4, 2001—3:23:00

67 Honolulu Marathon, December 9, 2001—3:48:34

68 Rome Marathon, March 24, 2002—3:49:38

69 Paris Marathon, April 7, 2002—3:52:43

70 Toronto Marathon, September 15, 2002—3:28:10

71 Portland Marathon, Oregon, October 6, 2002—3:38:00

72 Amsterdam Marathon, October 20, 2002—4:27:00

73 New York City Marathon, November 3, 2002—3:37:00

74 Marathon in the Parks, Maryland, November 17, 2002—3:57:21

75 Honolulu Marathon, December 8, 2002—3:47:29

76 Miami Tropical Marathon, February 2, 2003—3:16:16

77 Boston Marathon, April 14, 2003—3:22:00

78 Kona Marathon, June 21, 2003—5:21:00

79 Pikes Peak Marathon, Colorado, August 17, 2003—7:24:00

80 Médoc Marathon; Bordeaux, France, September 6, 2003—4:41:18

81 Wichita Marathon, Kansas, October 19, 2003—3:35:47

82 Auckland Marathon, New Zealand, November 2, 2003—3:39:00

83 Tulsa Marathon, November 22, 2003—3:28:00

84 Barbados Marathon, December 7, 2003—4:38:00

85 Hog Eye Marathon; Fayetteville, Arkansas, March 28, 2004—3:43:58

86 Boston Marathon, April 19, 2004—3:34:00

87 Vancouver International Marathon, British Columbia, May 2, 2004—3:25:43

88 Bunco Calgary Marathon, July 11, 2004—3:55:57

89 Mesa Falls Marathon; Ashton, Idaho, August 28, 2004—4:00:42

90 Des Moines Marathon, Iowa, October 17, 2004—3:20:34

91 Marine Corps Marathon, Washington, D.C., October 31, 2004—3:28:33

92 Marathon in the Parks; Montgomery County, Maryland, November 14, 2004—3:45:01

93 White Rock Marathon; Dallas, Texas, December 12, 2004—3:32:58

94 Las Vegas International Marathon, January 30, 2005—3:36:59

95 George Washington Birthday Marathon; Greenbelt, Maryland, February 20, 2005—3:49:40

96 Virginia Creeper, Abingdon, March 13, 2005—3:49:36

97 Ocean City Marathon; Ocean City, Maryland, April 16, 2005—3:53:00

98 Vancouver Marathon, British Columbia, May 1, 2005—3:57:19

99 Coventry Healthcare Delaware Marathon, Wilmington, May 15, 2005—3:35:07

100 Grandfather Mountain Marathon; Boone, North Carolina, July 9, 2005—3:46:00

Acknowledgments

To borrow a well-used phrase, it takes a village to publish a book, and I was lucky enough to have a particularly great bunch of villagers to help me turn this idea into a reality. First, thanks to my agent, Lauren Abramo, for her support and ever-helpful guidance. Thanks also to Bill Wolfsthal and Sarah Van Bonn at Skyhorse Publishing for their patience and vision, and to Jan Seeley and Rich Benyo of *Marathon & Beyond* for a decade's worth of friendship and encouragement. I still remember the first article query I sent over to Rich: I suggested a word limit, and he e-mailed back that I shouldn't worry about that; I should just write all that I needed to say. It's a freedom I've never taken for granted, and which I hope I haven't abused.

Thanks to Dave Harrell for being a big part of my story, and to Renata Carvalho for running and racing with me and for offering me valuable advice after reading the first draft of this book. Thanks also to my pace team organizers, who have invited me to enjoy a new side of marathoning: Josh Leibman of FunnerRunner and Marathon Memories, and Star and Darris Blackford and the entire Clif Bar Pace Team family.

Finally, a world of thanks to my sisters, Marlene and Dori, and their families, all my friends and colleagues, and especially to my parents, who I wish could have been here to see this.

About the Author

JEFF HOROWITZ is a certified personal trainer and running coach, living in Washington, D.C. He got hooked on marathoning in 1987, and in addition to his own running, he has coached hundreds of others to run their first marathon while raising money for various charities. When he's not busy doing these things, he's also an attorney, columnist, husband, and father to little Alex Michael, who pleased his daddy by quickly learning how to say, "Look, I'm running!" Visit Jeff at www.runtothefinishline.com.